THUNDER
on the RIGHT
The Protestant Fundamentalists

THUNDER
on the
RIGHT

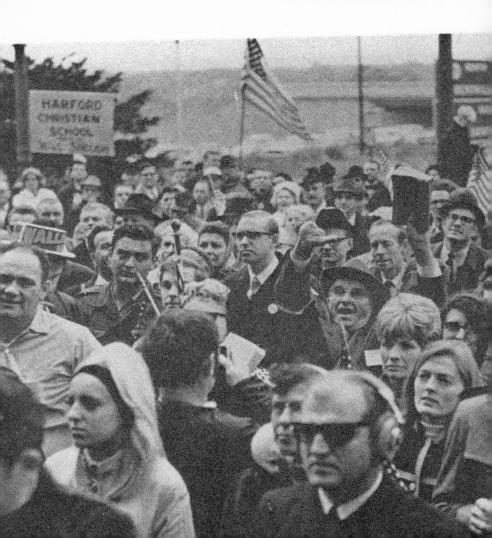

The Protestant Fundamentalists

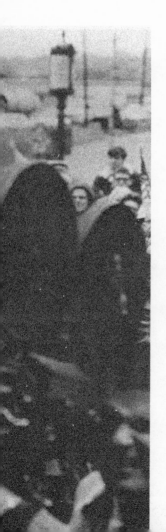

Gary K. Clabaugh

Nelson-Hall Company
nh Chicago

Library of Congress Cataloging in Publication Data

Clabaugh, Gary K.
  Thunder on the right

  Includes bibliographical references.
  1. Fundamentalism. 2. Radicalism—United States.
I. Title
BT82.2.C53   280'.4   74–9551
ISBN 0–88229–103–4

Contents

extension and McIntire's style of leadership. Hargis
points the way: *The "Twentieth Century Reformation
Hour" goes on the air.* Emergence of the contemporary
American Radical Right: *The blending.* Cape May
complex. ACCC's ouster of McIntire and other difficulties. Cape Canaveral complex. A last word.

Preface

Nine years ago I began my teaching career in a small town in south-central Pennsylvania. I was to teach geography to seventh graders. When I began my work I was determined, as only the naively new can be, to give the subject vitality and to avoid recapitulating the dreary recitations that had been called geography in my school days.

The challenge of such a change was not long in coming. My textbook, not of my own choosing of course, began with a description of the universe and our own solar system. As I recall, it commenced by saying, 'I'm sure you all have heard the lines, 'Twinkle, twinkle, little star. . . .' " This was the way that the authors had chosen to introduce the awe-inspiring wonders of the whirling enormity around us to adolescents who had cut their teeth on channel selectors. What followed was equally drab.

I was determined to get off on an interesting note. Consequently, I decided to begin by trying to communicate to the children some of the same kind of knowledge that had enabled me to experience a profound sense of my own minuteness as I looked into the blackness of the sky. This seemed a meaningful thing to me, albeit a small one in the totality of life, and I hoped that some of the students could be brought to share it with me.

Things went slowly at first; much more slowly than I had imagined during my absurdly optimistic planning sessions. But after I got over the initial shock of seeing how difficult my job was going to be, I became increasingly capable of interpreting small signs of success as positive reinforcement. (I have never been able to decide if this ability marked the beginning of pedagogical maturity or the commencement of self-delusion.) These small signs slowly became more numerous, and as they did, I began to feel that my ambition to teach had not been totally misplaced. To be sure, I had been naive about how easily one could become a good teacher, and I had badly underestimated the ability of the students to remain indifferent, but it still seemed a promising career.

The discussion of the nature of the universe and our solar system had been going on for better than a week when it began to catch hold. For some of the students the classes were becoming something more than "just plain schoolwork." The class discussions slowly became animated with real interest, and for the first time I found myself unrelieved when the bell signaled the end of the period.

Toward the end of the time I had allotted to this subject, a student asked a question that seemed to offer an ideal transition from the enormities of space and the more pedestrian aspects of our own earth that the study guide told me I must teach. We were in the midst of a discussion that seemed to be one of the best of the year when one of the students asked, with the sincerity that is best reserved for youth, "How did life begin? How did we start?" Other members of the class indicated that they wanted to know too. This was just too good an opportunity to miss. A natural transition from the introduction of our earth whirling in the universe to the phenomena on its surface.

While it was obviously opportune that it had worked out this way, there were grounds for apprehension. After all, the controversy surrounding the teaching of the theory of evolution had not died completely in rural America and the conservative nature of this community was legend, even among the school faculty. (They tended to regard such things as labor unions as vaguely un-

American.) But this was 1964, not 1925, and I had promised myself that I would not emasculate my teaching through moral cowardice. However, since this subject touched close to the quick of some of the people in the community, there was a need for scrupulous fairness and caution. I was also aware that this subject might do more harm than good amongst the more traditional of the youngsters if it were not handled with delicacy. With these cautions in mind I stumbled backwards, but with my eyes wide open, into a controversy which still evokes a strange mixture of humor and anger as it is recalled.

The subject of evolution was called to the fore by the nature of the student's question, but the way in which it was answered was my responsibility. I told them that I knew of three basic explanations of how life on earth began. One of these followed a literal interpretation of the Bible, one incorporated the general concept of evolution into a Biblical framework, and one was solely based on the scientific observations of man. I then read from Genesis, and told them that some people in our society felt that this was precisely how it happened, right down to the seven 24-hour days. I then proceeded to relate a simplified version of Darwin's theory, with current additions, and told them that some felt that this version alone was sufficient. Finally I related how many people did not feel that Darwin's observations were contradictory to the Bible, but rather only explained the events related in Genesis in detail. The whole telling was marked by discussion and obvious interest. No doubt about it, here was one subject that stirred them. I concluded by reminding the students that this subject had religious overtones and that I was unable to answer all of their questions because of my lack of religious training. For these answers I referred them to their own clergymen, a touch that seemed to give the whole thing elegance at the time.

Besides feeling a little silly about presenting the idea that life could have been created in seven 24-hour days as a credible notion, I felt really satisfied with what had taken place in my class that day. There had been genuine interest and animation on the part of most of the students, and it had been meaningful to me.

My first hint of impending trouble came with a final cigarette in the faculty room before going home. I related my interesting day to a group of three or four of the regulars. They seemed to feel that the ground traversed was most hazardous and that trouble might ensue. Since none of those present was noted for his courage or inventiveness, I put aside their comments as sour grapes and headed for home to relate the triumph, now bigger than life, to the wife.

On the way home I switched on the car radio, and tuned to the local "gospel" station that featured an "open mike" call-in show. This evening's show was different. It featured me. At least it featured a Satanic character who taught EVILution in the local seventh grade where prayer and Bible reading were banned by law. The more I listened to the callers and the "moderator" reviling this evil, the more I came to appreciate the full meaning of Charlie Brown's plaintive comment, "My stomach hurts." What made it even worse was that what I was hearing was, in the main, untrue. No mention was made of the scrupulous effort to present all sides, of the instructions, now suddenly important, to consult a minister if any religious questions troubled them; only the fact that the insidious, pro-Communist theory of evolution had made an inroad into our schools.

I thought of calling in myself and denouncing the charges as untrue. However, such a call might lend credence to the station's programming and to the topic at hand. Since the station was widely known as a forum for the "lunatic fringe," the principal's words, I believe, it seemed that the best course of action would be to ignore the broadcast. This was to prove impossible.

Following a restless night, I found myself with new courage in the morning. I had reevaluated everything taught the previous day and it still did not seem to be lacking. When I arrived at school it became obvious that I was not the only one who listened to this particular radio station. Most of my fellow teachers greeted me with that bemused look of expectation that is usually reserved for condemned men. They seemed to feel that I had made a serious blunder, and those who had warned me the night before now awaited vindication of their judgement with apparent relish. They did not have to wait long. A summons came that I was to report to the principal's office.

The conversation with the principal began on a fairly amiable note. He recounted that he had been tuned to the local radio station when THE subject had been raised. He added that he was fully cognizant of the irresponsible reputation of the radio station, and felt that the full truth had not been aired. I heaved an inaudible sigh of relief. BUT, he said, one not only had to be careful about what one said, but also about what one might be accused of saying. The rest of the conversation followed a similar vein and ended with his fatherly advice to lay off of this delicate subject. How long I should lay off was not clear but the distinct impression was communicated that forever would not be too long.

I must confess that I cannot recall the full conversation in detail, for I began stewing when the principal reminded me of the dangers lurking in what I didn't say, but might be accused of. It seemed obvious that if you talked about anything beyond the crushingly mundane, you could always be *accused* of impropriety. Slowly, against my better judgement, I found myself growing obdurate. I ended up righteously indignant and mad as hell. Rather quickly I found myself backed into a corner, refusing to recant, refusing to soft-pedal, and terribly confused. The circumstances I was involved in were absurd and the formless guilt that had been quietly wooing me was slowly turning into rage.

The story can be finished quickly and mercifully now, for the rest of it has the same slow but inevitable quality that dust has when it settles. Finding me reasonably civil, but unrepentant, the principal told me, in a voice that suggested that more was to come, that I could return to my duties. The rest of the day was misery. I continued to teach, more timidly now, on the same subject, but as I taught, I found myself spending a good deal of the time wondering which one of "them" had started the ugly scene. The spontaneity and enthusiasm were gone, replaced by anxiety and angry suspicion. As for the other teachers, they seemed to be drawing back from me, as if my troubles might be contagious.

That evening I could not resist turning on the radio again. The subject was still the same; although now some of my students had jumped, uninvited, into the turmoil. They were defending me but it only served to fuel the fires. I shut the radio off and tried to shut it out of my mind. The former was easy, the latter impossible.

The following morning the principal informed me that the Superintendent of Schools wished to see me after class. The time of the meeting served to swell my anxiety as the hours ticked by. The kids wanted to talk about the controversy. I wanted to quit.

The superintendent made me wait in his outer office; I got the uncomfortable feeling that I had been through this procedure before. However, the last time had been as a squirt-gunning highschooler about to face justice. The secretaries glanced at me as I sat in the seat normally reserved for adolescent offenders, then self-consciously looked away. Had this been a ceremony in humiliation it could not have been more effective.

When he finally consented to see me, the conversation with the superintendent was essentially the same as the one with the principal, with one interesting variation. It turned out that the superintendent's own son had been in my class, his name too common to have led me to make the connection. Thus the superintendent was at least partially aware of what had really taken place. A chance for vindication? Unfortunately, he too subscribed to the notion that my sin had been in touching at all on a subject that was prone to controversial misinterpretations. He was unmoved by the argument that the avoidance of everything significantly misinterpretable was the same thing as the avoidance of everything really meaningful. He listened politely, he even agreed to a point, but it did not change a thing. I remained civilly obdurate, but by this time my inner resolve was weakening. I had little heart for any more of this type of nonsense. Perhaps more courage would have remained had it not been fatally weakened by the paralysis of defense which comes from not really knowing your crime. The meeting ended inconclusively, but we both seemed to intuitively understand that a repeat of the deed was most unlikely.

Later, after some of my courage returned, I taught essentially the same thing. This time, however, I called it "natural selection." I did this on the theory that the trigger word "evolution" was the chief danger. It worked; no one seemed the wiser. Unfortunately, there was little joy in it. Making them wiser had been the whole idea. The *Funktionlust,* the joy of doing, was gone from teaching. Sometimes there was a halfhearted revival, but it was always dampened by the sour memory of that terrible beginning.

I later learned that this particular radio station was not just a voice for that "old time religion." On the contrary, it was a major mouthpiece for a variety of groups that I came to know as the Fundamental Protestant Radical Right. This station was the only one in the community. Indeed, due to the town's small size, it was the only public media of any type. Consequently, it had a power that even the most rational of local citizens had to recognize. While they would fully acknowledge the station's idiocy in private, they acted in public as if it broadcast a rational point of view. Thus, the station's smears, innuendos, and appeals to intolerance pervaded the community, giving it a neo-inquisitional quality. The local public schools—schools are hardly models of courage in any community—were reduced to paying intellectual ransom to the inquisitors. It was while living in this community, watching the public discourse dissolve under this assault and being assaulted myself, that my interest in the Fundamental Protestant Radical Right was formed.

These autobiographical comments, while serving to reveal the beginnings of my interest, also serve to point out a potential source of bias. Intimate involvement with the subject matter makes the already difficult task of objectivity more problematic. However, these incidents did occur, and it does not seem advisable to avoid the subject because of them. Consequently, the facts are related so that the reader may better judge for himself whether fairness and objectivity have been served in what follows.

If this personal experience were unique, or if it were typical of only this particular community, it would not count as a justification for studying the Fundamental Protestant Radical Right or its secular cousins. The fact is, however, that the experience is not uncommon, and the town not that much of an exception. On the contrary, the organizations loosely grouped under this classification are far more influential, both locally and nationally, than is commonly believed. Their resources are formidable. Their beliefs, while ridiculous, are so akin to Fascism that we ignore or laugh at them at our peril. Their actions are scurrilous and irresponsible. Proof of these contentions runs throughout this book.

Introduction

No compromise
no surrender

" **T**hose Germans who saw it all at the beginning—there were not very many; there never are, I suppose, anywhere—called Hitler the *Rattenfänger,* the "ratcatcher." Every American child has read *The Pied Piper of Hamlin.* Every German child has read it too. In German its title is *Der Rattenfänger von Hameln.*"[1]

Contemporary America also has its *Rattenfängers.* Some are identifiable through their public adulation of Hitler and Nazism. But the utter horror of this era of human history transforms these individuals into macabre political jokes.

There are other *Rattenfängers,* however who appear to be something else—Bible believing, freedom loving, fundamentalist preachers, for example. These individuals merit serious attention. After all, had the Pied Piper appeared to be what he really was, the rats of Hamlin would not have followed him to their death. Similarly, if the American public knows these *Rattenfängers* for what they are, they are unlikely to accept their invitations for a musical stroll.

The identification and detailed description of a portion of these political Pied Pipers—specifically that portion who drape themselves in the robes of Jesus Christ while frantically waving the American flag—is one function of this book. But if the "witch hunts" of the late Senator Joseph McCarthy taught us nothing else, they taught us that any identification of "the enemies within" must be accompanied by scrupulously documented evidence. Therefore, the central function of this book is to provide unimpeachable and exhaustive evidence that the movements described as threats to whatever tolerance and freedom we have are, in fact, just that.

Such evidence commonly comes in two varieties. The first involves the ideologies of the men and movements involved. If it can be established that these ideologies embody injustice, cruelty or fanatical irrationality, then we have reason to view them with alarm. What a man says he believes, however, and what his actions tell us he believes, can be different. Consequently, the second variety of evidence required before serious allegations are made is that these men or movements actually act consistent with their stated beliefs.

A number of books have portrayed the American Radical Right, including its religious segment, as a serious domestic threat. But they usually have done so by describing their ideologies rather than their actions. A unique feature of this work is that it provides detailed examples of their behavior as well as their ideologies. They are, it turns out, frighteningly consistent.

Ordinarily, the presence of a few *Rattenfängers* within the society is neither surprising nor particularly threatening—though we ignore them at our peril in even the most tranquil of times. But our times are far from tranquil; and as the tumult mounts, the Piper's tunes become more and more beguiling. Most ominously, our own government sounds more and more in tune with the Pipers. Consider the Presidential statements that later were "rendered inoperative," or the government-sponsored burglaries, domestic espionage, "enemy lists," and various other "White House Horrors" unraveled by the Senate Select Committee on Watergate. Ponder the "secret" bombings of Cambodia that were obviously no secret to the individuals being bombed but were kept quite secret from the American people for reasons of "national security." Consider what might yet be revealed, then ponder this quote from Milton Mayer's book describing life in Nazi Germany, titled, *They*

Thought They Were Free. It was published nearly twenty years ago. A German who survived it, describes it.

> What happened here was the gradual habituation of the people, little by little, to being governed by surprise; to receiving decisions deliberated in secret; to believing that the situation was so complicated that the government had to act on information which the people could not understand, or so dangerous that, even if the people could understand it, it could not be released because of national security. And their sense of identification with Hitler, their trust in him, made it easier to widen this gap and reassured those who would have otherwise worried about it.
>
> This separation of government from people, this widening of the gap, took place so gradually and so insensibly, each step disguised (perhaps not even intentionally) as a temporary measure or associated with true patriotic allegiance or with real social purposes. And all the crises and reforms (real reforms too) so occupied the people that they did not see the slow motion underneath, of the whole process of government growing remoter and remoter."[2]

We should remember that the process described above began long before Hitler and Nazism were even newsworthy. Indeed it seems quite unlikely that the Third Reich would have even been possible had this not been the case.

Since a similar process is recognizable in contemporary America, it is both prudent and timely to scrutinize our own collection of *Rattenfängers* now.

While most volumes dealing with these individuals and movements treat their secular components in greatest detail, this book examines their fundamental Protestant portion most closely. This is done for several reasoins. First, when examining this particular portion of the American Radical Right we find considerable substantiation of historian Richard Hofstadter's contention that our own domestic Radical Right can be explained as an extension of the "fundamentalist style of mind."[3] Consequently, any in-depth understanding of the entire movement requires a detailed background on its fundamentalist portion. Second, since deference has traditionally been shown to men of the cloth or to beliefs which are essentially religious, the men and movements described in this book have sometimes escaped the degree of scrutiny to which secular organizations, such as the John Birch Society, have been subjected. This volume pays no such deference.

The book attends to historical background, ideology, leaders, organizations, resources, methods, and impact on our contemporary culture. It is intended to provide anyone with a serious interest in America's Radical Right—particularly its fundamentalist portion, which includes Carl McIntire, Billy James Hargis, Edgar Bundy, and others—with in-depth understanding. Additionally, the book is organized in such a fashion that individuals with particular interests, Carl McIntire's history, for example, can readily find the facts.

It should also be noted that much of the data on the actions of these individuals and movements was derived from several controversies involving public education—most notably the sex education controversy of the late 1960s. Therefore this volume is particularly useful to those who have a special interest in the Radical Right's ability to influence the process of schooling.

Finally, although serious purpose characterizes this book, I have adopted Bertrand Russell's advice that ". . .those who are solemn and pontifical are not to be successfully fought by being even more solemn and even more pontifical." Therefore, I have permitted some of the black humor I see in this to surface.

section 1

The Fundradists in action: The sex education controversy of the 1960s

Most Americans have, in one way or another, encountered the Fundamental Protestant Radical Right. Some have had their lives altered in the process. Yet few recognize the chilling qualities of those they have encountered.

The nature of Protestantism is schismatic. Over the centuries it has divided and subdivided into thousands of sects and denominations. One consequence of this has been a blurring of the lines that separate its more responsible or conventional elements from its extremist fringe. For example, one might live next door to a church which has advocated an unprovoked nuclear attack on the Soviet Union in the name of Christ and country, or which teaches that Americans are God's one and only chosen people, and remain totally ignorant of this curious situation.[1] After all, it is like any other church when viewed from the outside.

Misidentification

The difficulty of isolating this extremist fringe is also attributable to the fact that a substantial portion of the news media ignores the political extremism of the Fundamental Protestant Radical Right by referring to them as "Fundamentalists." (Hereafter we will refer to the Fundamental Protestant Radical Right as Fundradists, for convenience.) For example, "Fundamentalist Preacher Carl McIntire predicted yesterday that 2,000 to 3,000 persons will join in a protest against. . .Soviet Leader Leonid I. Brezhnev."[2] Such reporting encourages the casually informed to regard Carl McIntire, Billy James Hargis, Edgar Bundy, and the others who share their ideology as a part of the common run of Fundamentalist Preachers. They are not. In fact, we shall see that the nature of their ideology causes them to be regarded as outcasts by the Fundamentalist mainstream. But misidentification still serves to legitimize them.

The cover of absurdity

Should anyone who still cherishes the hope that man is more or less rational happen to penetrate the shield of respectability afforded by the misidentification of the Fundradists, they may ignore or even laugh at what they discover. After all, it is utter nonsense to dogmatically maintain, as the Fundradists do, that God *needs* America and laissez-faire capitalism, or that all in the world is either good or evil and that the United States is the God-anointed champion of the goodness. This inanity leads otherwise learned men to regard them as unworthy of serious thought or prolonged attention. However, such an attitude inadvertently provides protection for those who would destroy the very tolerance that makes learned men possible.

Dogmatic devotion to intellectual rubbish has propelled more horror than we can catalogue. For instance, it was obvious and utter nonsense to maintain that all of Germany's woes were attributable to Jews, or to preach that "Nordic types" were supermen. Yet their childish prattle prompted "civilized" men to commit crimes against humanity that we, who did not witness the "final solution," cannot even imagine. Clearly, if this one glimpse into the Apocalypse taught us nothing else it taught us that one should not confuse the absence of intellectual substance with the absence of importance.

1

The Fundradists:
Placing them in context

Resources and organizations

G iven their misidentification as religious rustics and the related obscure obsurdity of their views, it is quite natural to imagine that the Fundamental Protestant Radical Right has minimal resources. Nothing could be further from the truth. In fact, if we take the combined budgets of just two of the largest of these organizations, Carl McIntire's "Twentieth Century Reformation" and Billy James Hargis' "Christian Crusade," we get an annual total of approximately $5 million.[1] In addition, McIntire's "Twentieth Century Reformation Hour" radio broadcast is heard over hundreds of radio stations five days a week, while Hargis' message beams out from an additional 100. In a new departure, Hargis also broadcasts weekly in "living color" over 40 television stations.[2]

Reverend McIntire's activities include the operation of two colleges, the "Beach Plum Restaurant" and the three largest resort hotels in Cape May, New Jersey, a weekly newspaper with a circulation of over 120,000, a 1,800 member Bible Presbyterian Church in Collingswood, New Jersey, the Presidency of the Bible Presbyterian Synod, the Presidency of the International Council of Christian Churches, an international relief organization, inter-

3

national and domestic missionary organizations, an orphanage, Faith Theological Seminary in Elkins Park, Pennsylvania, involvement in the operation of a radio station which was recently denied license renewal for violating the "Fairness Doctrine," and a newly formed recording company.[3] Recently he also acquired the Cape Kennedy Hilton, which is only five years old, and an added assortment of Florida real estate that included office buildings and condominium apartments in the vicinity of Cape Canaveral. The value of this deal has been estimated at between $4 and $25 million. McIntire also temporarily went to sea with a "pirate" radio station when the operating license of his station was not renewed. He was torpedoed by a court order. The Rev. Hargis' activities, while not quite so diversified, are equally imposing. They will be outlined in detail in a later chapter.

It is readily apparent that the Fundamental Protestant Radical Right (hereafter referred to as the Fundradists for convenience) is hardly a bushleague operation confined to decrepit Gospel halls in the hinterlands. On the contrary, the movement is characterized by multimillion-dollar budgets, extensive real estate holdings, computerized contributor lists, international radio broadcasts, several television shows, resort hotels, schools, and colleges, publishing houses, recording companies, endorsement by governors, U.S. Senators, and foreign heads of state, handsome expense accounts, and jet trips around the world.[4] Obviously, the derisive laughter often directed at them is not justified on the basis of any lack of material substance. In fact, the entire Radical Right is a force that our society must reckon with and the Fundamental Protestant wing is a major portion thereof. This wing is all the more significant because of its religious trappings. By wrapping themselves in the flag, the Radical Right have been able to forestall much of the criticism that might have been directed at them. The Bible, and a "Reverend" before one's name, add greatly to this protective coloration.

Evidence of influence

It has been established that the Fundradists are a significant component of our society in terms of their resources. It remains

to be shown whether they have any real influence. It is not difficult
to find such evidence. In examining the Radical Right's positions
and programs, one is not long in discovering that a large portion
of their time, energy, and resouces are utilized in matters relating
to the public schools. This is particularly true of the Fundamental
Protestant portion. They concentrate their efforts on those areas
of schooling that are the most controversial and emotion-laden.
Some of the major issues in which they are heavily involved include: returning prayer and Bible reading to the public schools,
opposing Federal aid to education, trying to prevent busing, extolling the virtues of "freedom of choice," attacking "progressivism," "Words in Color," the "New Math," and other curriculum
innovations, and launching a vitriolic campaign against sex education and sensitivity training. Indeed, the last area mentioned,
that of sex education and sensitivity training, has been turned into
a major area of educational conflict on a national scale, due, in
large part, to their efforts.

The anti–sex education campaign

As a matter of fact, Hargis' Christian Crusade has been one of
the most vocal and effective opponents that either of these programs has had. In 1969 he launched a nationwide movement to
eradicate both. Hargis and many members of his staff toured the
country speaking in as many as four or five communities in a
week. Their campaign was characterized by emotionalism and by
charges which were, to put it mildly, highly controversial. The
general tone of the campaign, which abounded in charges of dis-
loyalty, subversion, and the basest of motives, is revealed in the
titles of some of the books sold at these gatherings by the Hargis
staff. They included: *Is the School House the Proper Place to
Teach Raw Sex?* by the now departed "Educational Director" of
the Crusade, Dr. Gordon Drake, *Sensitivity Training: Attack on
Christian Values and American Culture,* and *Blackboard Power:
NEA Threat to America,* both also by Drake. The last volume
proclaims on its cover: "WE ARE LOSING CONTROL OF
OUR SCHOOLS—POWER HUNGRY NEA LEADERS USE
TACTICS OF THE GOON—ENCOURAGE STRIKES,

THREATEN THE COMMUNITY WITH VIOLENCE—THE
NEA IS PROMOTING COMMUNIST CAUSES. OUR CHIL-
DREN ARE BEING INDOCTRINATED FOR A NEW COL-
LECTIVIST WORLD GOVERNMENT." Dr. Drake does not
have a gift for understatement.[5]

SIECUS. One of the primary thrusts of the Hargis campaign was
against the Sex Information and Education Council of the United
States (SIECUS). Members of the Council were accused of a
multitude of transgressions, and made into the arch-villains of
the piece. At their best they were portrayed to be bumbling,
lascivious incompetents; at worst, a sinister part of a subversive
plot to undermine the morality of the nation.

Hargis was joined in his assault on sex education and SIECUS
by the John Birch Society. The Society arrived on the scene of
the conflict a little late, but made up for this by the vehemence
of its attacks. SIECUS was also its favorite target. Soon, the
majority of rest of the Right joined in the fray.[6]

The distrust and fright that the Hargis entourage left in their
wake were astonishing. Parents are notoriously sensitive about
the welfare of their children, and rightfully so, but the tenor of the
attacks stirred many to hasty, and sometimes extreme, action.[7]
Certainly, sex education is controversial, and the arguments
against school involvement in it are many and often sound. Unfortunately, discussion of these real issues often became impossible because of the acrimony that the Fundradists and their
secular brethren left in their wake. Dialogue has a way of breaking
down when emotions reach a peak. This is especially so when the
fertile ground of the debate is sown with accusations of subversion,
pro-Communism, and immorality.

THE MEDIA'S RESPONSE. The Radical Right's assault on sex
education and sensitivity training did not go unnoticed by the
general public. On the contrary, it was belatedly detailed in
popular magazines such as *Look, Life, Redbook,* the *Reader's
Digest,* and many others.[8] These articles served to alert many

Americans to the fact that extremist organizations such as Hargis' Crusade could have a very real influence on the schools of the nation. It also raised another question that has yet to be answered. If the Radical Right, led by its Fundamental Protestant wing, could mount such a successful assault on educational programs, what might they be able to accomplish outside of the pedagogical realm?

THE OUTCOME. When the results of the Radical Right's assaults on sex education and sensitivity training are tallied, it is difficult to remain unimpressed. As of 1970, two State boards of education had taken action specifically opposing the Sex Information and Education Council of the United States. In addition, thirteen State legislatures had canceled, curtailed, or postponed their sex education programs; twenty others were considering investigating, restricting, or prohibiting theirs. In at least six States, citizens' groups had gone to court to keep sex education out of the schools.[9] Sensitivity training managed to avoid most of these thrusts. This was due, in part at least, to its comparative newness, uncertain identity, and relative scarcity. However, there can be little doubt that it has also suffered a setback.

The controversy withered somewhat in the waning weeks of the 1969–70 school year. This was due, in part at least, to the nearness of the summer vacation and to the eruption of major violence on the nation's college campuses, which drew the more immediate attention of the right. However, it is most unlikely that an issue which has proved so successful in recruiting new contributors and in exercising newfound muscle will be summarily abandoned. Periodic revivals should be expected. Moreover, the Fundradists now know that educational issues have real promise.

The role of the Fundamental Protestant Radical Right in the sex education and sensitivity training controversy clearly attests to the fact that the Fundradists do have a significant influence on American society. It also demonstrates their method of operation and its consequence. We will examine the controversy in detail in the next three chapters.

The issue of freedom

The sex education and sensitivity training controversy also illustrates a much larger issue in which the Fundamental Protestant
Radical Right is very much involved. This is the issue of freedom
itself—the foundation of democracy. Freedom is an imprecise
concept, the meaning of which tends to vary with the user, and
the specific situation involved. Nevertheless, the basic notion is
that human beings must be permitted to do what they wish so
long as they do not harm others, and that they must be able to
do this without fear. This ideal is not commonplace in reality.
In general, our society has come to tacitly recognize certain limits
to this fredom. For example, there is a decided difference in the
amount of freedom granted in the economic sector as opposed to
the political one.

Most importantly, although many of our freedoms are based on
law, they ultimately depend on fragile things such as tradition,
tacit agreement, and what we call "common decency."

THE THREAT TO FREEDOM.   Tradition, tacit agreements, and
"common decency" are adequate in a society where each contend-
ing side listens to the other's arguments, assumes the good will of
all concerned, and acts in a responsible fashion. Unfortunately,
the Radical Right, including its Fundamental Protestant component, does not adhere to these rules. They view the world as
being essentially dichotomous, with no middle ground. You are
either for America—their version of it, that is—or you are, at best,
a misguided fool; at worst, a traitor. You are either on the side of
"light and of Christ," or on the side of "darkness, compromise,
and the Devil."[10] Given this world view, the question of freedom
becomes nonsense. Open discussion of controversial ideas is error
or subversion. There are no legitimate alternatives to their pre-
conceptions.

There are two basic dimensions to freedom, and the Fundamental Protestant Radical Right is involved in both of them. First,
freedom involves restraints that might be placed on individuals
from without in the form of restrictive laws or regulations. An in-

teresting example of this type of restraint would be the various State laws against abortion that were recently nullified by the U.S. Supreme Court. The Radical Right is deeply involved in trying to retain those that exist and adding new ones. The second dimension involves restraints which are self-imposed by individuals themselves. By avoiding controversial matters which might make one the subject of social pressure the individual can impose a limitation on his own freedom that goes far beyond that which any restrictive law could hope to accomplish.

It is this type of restriction of freedom that the Radical Right is most deeply involved in. They are quite willing to label anyone who departs from the narrowest conception of yesterday's conventional wisdom as a "vicious underminer of youth," as a "disseminator of UNESCO propaganda," a "pro-Red," or a "user of children as pawns." Indeed, the range of uncomplimentary adjectives that they use with abandon boggles the mind.[11] When these charges are fed to a community that has been reared on a steady diet of anti-Communism as American credo, and that is terribly distraught over the present confusing state of things, they can create an atmosphere of insecurity that forces a compliance with extralegal limits on freedom that effectively strangles it. And, perhaps most ironically, this type of insecurity even touches those who really do endorse the narrowest conception of yesterday's conventional wisdom. Because of the irresponsible way in which charges are hurled about, even they cannot be certain that they are clean. Thus they become victims of the same nagging uncertainty that they were willing to see inflicted on others.[12]

THE INDUCEMENT OF SOCIAL PARALYSIS. It is easy to see that the more individuals concern themselves with the kind of social, economic, political, and ethical questions that really matter, the more vulnerable they will be to the kind of attacks on freedom that emanate from the Radical Right. On the other hand, those kinds of issues are precisely the ones which are most urgent. Consequently, we are presented with a classic conflict situation. The more meaningful an individual's actions become, the more vulnerable he is to vitriolic attacks from a Radical Right that has proved unconscionable in the past. On the other hand, the more irrelevant the individual's participation in society is or becomes, the less chance society has of ever solving its basic problems. Social paralysis sets in.

There is no easy solution to this dilemma. No matter what course a man chooses, there will be penalties. Furthermore, given the present state of affairs, it is not the kind of decision that can be indefinitely postponed. One thing is certain, however, and this is that American citizens will have to summon the power and courage necessary to face the Radical Right if our society is to deal with the major issues of the latter half of this century.

The presence of the Fundamental Protestant segment of the Radical Right is going to make this task all the more problematic. American society breeds a great reluctance to attack churches or men of the cloth. Whether or not the Fundamental Protestant Radical Right merits this kind of genteel circumspection will be left for the reader to judge. But, however the case may be decided, this Fundamentalist contingent at least begins any conflict with this factor in its favor.

The emergence of pluralism

The autobiographical experience in the Preface, the sex education and sensitivity training struggle, and the more general problems relating to freedom, while hardly an exhaustive list, do serve to furnish very real illustrations of the way in which the entire Radical Right is involved in the general affairs of the nation. However, there is one specific area of public policy that is of special concern to the Fundamental Protestant Radical Right. This involves the matter of the proper relationship of religion and the state. Until the first years of the nineteenth century, this nation was not only Christian, but decidedly Protestant. The great influx of immigrants into America that began in the first half of the nineteenth century marked the end of what had been essentially an Anglo-Saxon, Protestant culture. As American culture became more pluralistic, there was a gradual diminuation of Anglo-Saxon, Protestant domination. While the nation still embraced a broadly Christian position, it became increasingly capable of avoiding intra-Christian doctrinal controversy.

By the time the twentieth century was well along, many of the blatantly religious restrictions had been eliminated from public life. This was necessitated by the fact that the public was no longer homogeneous in its religious beliefs. The process began as one of broadening the base of Protestants by including Catholics. Then it involved the addition of numerous individuals who are either not Christian or just not religious in any formalistic sense.

This gradual dereligionizing of society was dramatically illustrated in 1963. In this year the Supreme Court ruled that religious proceedings of any kind in the public schools are unconstitutional. The court maintained that this type of proceeding tended to "coerce" children into taking part, thus violating the First Amendment's prohibition against governmental "establishment of religion." We need not review the controversy that has been stirred by this decision. Suffice it to say that the ban on prayer and Bible reading did not receive great popular support. Numerous communities openly defied the law, and citizen groups sprang up around the country, circulating petitions, and attempting to have the ruling overcome.[13]

The fertile ground

Today the country is in a period of great turmoil and self-doubt. Values, norms, and institutions are being challenged, attacked, and defied. Many Americans feel threatened. They are alarmed and dismayed and look for an explanation of the trend. Some have come to feel that such simplistic things as the loss of prayer and Bible reading in the public schools has caused what they perceive as national decay. Similarly simplistic explanations serve as reasons for the youth rebellion, crime, drugs, welfare, high taxes, inflation, and almost everything else they feel angry about.[14]

Such a situation is fertile ground for the Fundamental Protestant Radical Right. Claiming to be the inheritors and preservers of the Christian-American tradition, they have seized this confusion and exploited it. Portraying themselves as the heroic leaders of

the movement to save "our Christian nation" from "Godless, atheistic Communism," and proclaiming themselves as the only "real
Americans," the Fundamental Protestant Radical Right is constantly searching for causes that rival sex education in their
popular appeal.

The disloyal opposition

While it would be most inadvisable to say that American citizens
do not have every right to join in public debates, like the one
concerning prayer and Bible reading or sex education in the
schools, it is the manner in which the Fundamental Protestant
Radical Right does so that is significant. As was suggested earlier,
they do not constitute a loyal opposition that is just one more
part of civic debate. On the contrary, by accusing those who disagree with them of being "un-American," "dupes of the international Communist conspiracy," "agents of Satan," and the like,
they serve to break down the kind of responsible discussion a
democracy must have if it is to survive.

As has been shown, there was a time, as the Fundamental Right
claims, when the nation was tied very closely to a relatively conservative brand of Protestant Christianity. But, as was pointed
out, those were far different times. To insist that the country's
troubles can be remedied by a return to these ostensibly simpler
times, which the Fundradists mythologize as a golden age of
theocracy, is to insist on the impossible. However, the suggestion
still has powerful emotional appeal to those who feel pressed
against the wall by modern trends. Through their irresponsible
accusations and dichotomous pronouncements the Fundamental
Protestant Radical Right feeds and exploits this pressure, thus
accelerating a polarization that already threatens to tear the nation
apart.

Thus we see that the educational issues, such as prayer and Bible
reading or sex education in the schools, come to blend imperceptibly into more general issues. Since the very early sixties the
Radical Right has been spending many millions of dollars in an
effort to influence broad national public policy and opinion. True

Now — leave in
Office — have
finished —

```
                                        CA
                          77  EMP  MDSE
                     7245289       1.00+*
                        20502      1.00+S
                     4.000% TAX     .04+
              6457      20502      1.04+S
              6457      20502      1.04+T
              6457    1 26 79
```

to the form that they display in their activities directed at the schools, these efforts have been characterized by the dissemination of fright and distrust of basic American institutions and values.[15] What Dr. Franklin Littel calls "the politics of the end time"[16] seeps, like spilled talc, into every cranny of national life. By examining their influence on education, as we will in the next several chapters, noneducators can gain some appreciation of what this seepage could mean.

Anti-Communism as American credo

Fifty or more years of national anxiety about Communism has created a beneficent environment for the Radical Right. They are warily tolerated with the same kind of inverse logic that led many well-meaning liberals of the thirties into an uneasy compromise with Stalinism. It is a complex and frustrating world, and living in it exposes one to a terrible temptation to explain the particularly troubling portions of it away with visions of an underlying Communist conspiracy. In fact, it is so tempting and so common that facetious reference to such an explanation of an event, while in literate company, is sure to generate some mirth. Therein lies another rub!

There *is* something comic about Red-hating, "patriotic" Americans who see card-carrying Communists everywhere that I.Q. exceeds foot size. This is liberally attested to by literary efforts, such as *Dr. Strangelove,* that have poked successful fun in this direction. There is, however, a nervous quality in this humor that reveals its origin in the jugular vein. All too frequently, however, the nervousness is concealed by civil inattention and the humor tends to divert attention from the very real power of the Radical Right and from the basis for the nervous quality of the humor. The fact is that when a significant component of a nation's population will tolerate no ambiguities, no equivocations, no reservations, and which is determined to squelch every challenge to this position, it just is not a suitable basis for unqualified comedy. Those "little old ladies in tennis shoes" screeching "Commie!" are usually funniest when you are not the one they are screeching at. This is particularly true in America, where it is all too common an occurrence to have otherwise responsible citizens equating pro-Communism with any significant departure from conformity.

The Radical Right has its greatest success in local communities, chiefly in intimidating the school system and an occasional library.[17] It is here in this microcosmic version of America that we can catch a glimpse of what awaits if their influence grows. And as the tide of distrust and discontent mounts ever higher, and as the residents of "middle America" become increasingly distraught, the danger of such growth becomes greater.

Many writers have pointed out the similarities between current domestic events and the events that preceded the rise of the Fascists in Italy and the Nazis in Germany. While such comparisons may be overdrawn, they are at least tentatively plausible. A thorough examination of the Fundamental Protestant Radical Right's activities in the sex education controversy, which follows, can furnish relevant data to help us decide how plausible.

Limitations

Why limit the effort to the Fundamental Protestant segment of the Radical Right? We will see that the "fundamental style" is present throughout the entire Radical Right. We will also see that membership in one blends into membership in the other, and that they both use common resources, materials, and methods. However, as has been pointed out, the Fundradists' claims to religious status has afforded protective coloration to those who twist the cross into a more ominous shape. What follows permits the reader to penetrate that camouflage and see what is being done in the name of God and country.

2

The changing wind

We have contended that men like Carl McIntire or Billy James Hargis are either unknown, thought of as rather ordinary "men of the cloth" who happen to lead curiously conservative and highly patriotic movements, or as harmless manifestations of absurdity, and that such misinformation and / or ignorance vastly increases their power. As the example of sex education clearly shows, such ignorance is anything *but* bliss when the Fundradists put on the pressure.

We also argued that the organizations we have classified as Fundradists, in conjunction with their brethren in the secular Radical Right, have a considerable impact on public education across America—especially when unusually sensitive subjects or issues are involved.

Several examples of this impact were cited in Chapter 1. Among them are the Fundradist efforts to return prayer and Bible reading to the public schools, to prevent "busing" and other desegregation moves, to snuff out the influences of "progressivism" and "permissiveness," and to oppose nearly every effort at curriculum reform that transcends a return to the "three R's" or *McGuffey's Eclectic Reader*.

Selections of the example

But the example providing the best, if roughhewn, paradigm of the Fundradists' ability to pressure the public schools is the still-simmering controversy over sex education. It is the purpose of this chapter to examine the origins of this controversy in detail.

Due to the unusually volatile nature of sex education, the Fundradists' impact on public schooling has been magnified. Obviously, had the issue centered on more mundane matters, their ability to generate pressure would have been lessened. Thus, in this sense at least, the controversy over sex education gives us an exaggerated view. But it is essential to remember that virtually any major changes in the policies and practices of the nation's public schools are bound to generate considerable volatility. One simply does not alter the lives of other people's children without evoking considerable and justifiable concern. Consequently, the "magnification" spoken of previously may not be as great as a superficial appraisal would suggest—especially in view of the fact that the current crisis in our schools must surely force *major* changes on our process of schooling if it is to survive. Further, it should be noted that as early as 1965 a Gallup poll revealed that seventy percent of the public approved of sex education in school. Thus this particular educational change was backed by a large majority of Americans. Obviously, the same thing could *not* be said of the many other major changes that necessity seems to dictate for our schools.

The origins of the controversy

The first tremblings that hinted of the impending furor over sex education were felt early in 1968. They came, appropriately enough, from Billy James Hargis' Tulsa-based Christian Crusade.[1] Prior to 1968, Hargis, the leading Fundradist organizer in terms of income, had made periodic attacks on certain aspects of American education. Usually these attacks focused on "permissivism," John Dewey, "progressivism," or, curiously, the rising "threat" of the National Education Association. But these attacks were episodic and were usually made in conjunction with some other issue. The only time Hargis and his organization really involved themselves with public schooling in any concerted way prior to 1968 was in 1964 when Hargis actively supported the Becker Amendment to put prayer and Bible reading back in schools. This effort temporarily cost him his tax-exempt status.[2]

Dr. Gordon V. Drake

The beginning of the "Christian Crusade's" utilization of the state of public schooling as one of its most successful auxiliary issues can be traced to Hargis' employment of Dr. Gordon V. Drake as the "Director" of the Crusade's newly formed "Department of Education." Drake was hired by Hargis in January of 1968—rudely interrupting his third year as Dean of Carl McIntire's Shelton College.

Unlike most Fundradists, Drake holds an *earned* doctorate in higher education and administration from the University of Denver. Before joining Hargis' "Crusade," he was a teacher in the public schools of Washington and Arizona; taught at Wisconsin State University, where he was fired for allegedly injecting Radical Rightist propaganda into his assignments and "aiding enemies of the college,"[3] served as an educational administrator in Hong Kong for one year, and put in two and one-half years as Dean of McIntire's Shelton College. Drake also wrote for the Birch Society magazine, *American Opinion,* from 1966 to 1968.[4]

The general assault on public education begins

Just two months after Drake joined the "Crusade" staff a series of messages were begun over Hargis' radio network attacking the state of public education. The first of these attacks was aired over Hargis' broadcast network on March 2, 1968, and was delivered by Hargis himself. It concerned Dr. Caleb Gattegno's reading method, Words in Color. Beginning his criticism with the claim that Dr. Gattegno allegedly developed this method while working

for UNESCO, Hargis proceeded to charge that the method utilized
a "sick vocabulary" that was also ". . .a good, solid revolutionary
vocabulary of which Stokely Carmichael could be proud."[5] Hargis
then argued that one of the method's readers, *Book of Stories,*
"makes a subtle attack on the family," and then finished his broadcast by castigating the method on the grounds that the experiences
contained within it were deliberately designed to be equally applicable to all English-speaking learners. This Hargis equated with
starting " 'one worldism' in the first grade."[6]

Hargis made no mention of Drake in this broadcast—a rather
curious fact when one discovers that a slightly expanded version
of Hargis' broadcast, with many paragraphs containing identical
wording, was published that summer in Dr. Gordon V. Drake's
book *Blackbeard Power: NEA Threat to America.*[7]

Any doubt as to the identity of the architect of Hargis' use of
education as a major auxiliary cause was dispelled the following
week when Drake himself took the Crusade microphone. His first
and second broadcasts dealt with the sinister threat posed by the
growing militancy of the National Education Association. Drake
charged that this was evidence that "The NEA seeks to control
the entire educational scene, and it will, if it has its way, produce
a new socialistic society for America."[8] He then went on to suggest the inevitable conspiracy, a theme common to all of the
Radical Right, by alleging that "The American public simply does
not realize what the hierarchy is really up to."[9] They were, Drake
proclaimed, in the act of "taking over education" by working
"hand in glove with the Federal government."[10]

As the week drew to a close Drake's attacks on public education
grew rougher. Now he was verbally lashing out with descriptions
of how, "while good men slept. . .others had sawed the legs off
their beds, and (given) the progressivists, such as John Dewey, the
opportunity to indoctrinate literally thousands of teachers and administrators."[11] And he backed these thrusts with others that
linked the alleged "leg sawing" to sexual perversion, Darwinism,
and the unrest that was then gripping many of the nation's college
campuses—a curious but compelling combination.[12]

In the final minutes of his first week of broadcasting Drake also left some footprints on the face of racial justice by denouncing the U.S. Office of Education's desire to promote a "cultural mix" in the nation's schools:

> What is this cutural mix? Well they are going to mix the good with the bad; the high with the low; the wealthy with the poor; the Negro with the Puerto Rican, the Spanish American, the Jew, the Irish. All well and good! However, proposals of this sort often tend to pull down the better elements of society to a common denominator rather than pull up the poorer elements. You can't mix bad with good and have anything but a wishy washy gray as a result. In other words, a basic principle of physics is completely ignored by the social planners, of which Harold Howe is a leader in America today.[13]

On Monday and Tuesday of the following week the attacks on public education continued with Drake still at the microphone. Now, however, it was the Encyclopaedia Britannica's *Junior Edition Literature Sampler* which was "spoonfeeding subversion to the innocents."[14] The entire broadcast series ended with the following admonition:

> May we humbly suggest that parents keep a watchful eye on what their children read. Find out who the authors are. Find out their backgrounds. Maybe a little censorship at this time is a good thing. It is our duty as Christian and American parents!

Drake's series of broadcasts on the "Crises in American Schools" closed without any mention of the issue of sex education. In fact, that issue went unmentioned for an additional three months. But the general tactic was apparent. Drake's new position within the "Crusade" signaled the beginning of an attempt by Hargis to use the state of American education as an auxiliary cause of major proportions. He was, however, not destined to hit real "pay dirt" until the summer of 1968.

Less than two weeks after Drake's series of broadcasts, the *Weekly Crusader* featured an article by him entitled "Blackboard Power NEA—Threat to America." This feature promoted Drake's "forthcoming book by the same title."[15] The relationship of this article to the impending furor over sex education is not direct.

But when the book appeared late in the summer of 1968, all of chapter 10 was devoted to a scathing criticism of sex education and contained virtually all of the basic components of the Fundradists' assault on the various types of courses that attempted to deal with this delicate subject.[16] Thus, if Drake and Hargis were not aware of the potentialities of the sex education issue in March (and one is hard pressed to explain why, if they *were* aware of it, they failed to use it) they obviously learned of its existence sometime in the spring of 1968. But there are some interesting possibilities. First, in response to general social upheavals and resultant changes of sexual mores, there have been all sorts of advocates for public school sex education since the turn of the century. So it was hardly a new idea.[17] For the most part, however, these appeals fell on deaf or outraged ears. Their time had not yet come.

By the mid-1960s, however, many Americans, probably impelled by the growing upheaval in values that characterized the times, had begun to press for some sort of public schooling that dealt with the "facts of life." What they wanted varied widely. In retrospect, perhaps too widely. But they clearly sensed a need for some sort of instruction that would, in some way or other, grapple with the newly emerging "counterculture" and the "new morality" that was its pulse.[18]

Clearly, more and more young people were either not listening to the advice or commands of their parents, or were getting no sex education at home and were "doing their own thing." So, virtually by default, the public schools were elected to try either to erect a bridge across this particular generation gap and restore some semblance of order and coherence to the nation's sexual mores or, at the very least, to keep these young people free from venereal disease and unwanted pregnancies.

Thus a *grass roots* demand for action propelled an ill-prepared public school system into one of the most important curriculum changes of the decade. Of course, this issue was fraught with dozens of pitfalls and snares capable of entrapping even the most cautious. And it did just that.

GRASS ROOTS OPPOSITION: THE OPENING WEDGE. Thus this explosive issue was forced to the surface by a public demand engendered by a fundamental social change. But the Radical Right, usually closely attuned to matters of this sort, completely over-looked sex eductaion's potential as an auxiliary cause until grass roots opposition at the local level caused them to redirect their attention. Once they did, however, they lost little time in pursuing the matter with passion.

The importance of Frank A. Capell

The abundance of Radical Rightist groups and individual activists in this nation—there were 3,406 separate entries in the 1965 (fifth) edition of the Alert American's Association's *First National Directory of "Rightist" Groups, Publications and Some Individuals in The United States (and Some Foreign Countries)*[19]— makes it impossible to determine precisely which Radical Rightists were the first to recognize the potentialities of this issue. But the first *to be noticed* was Frank A. Capell. And it was opposition of the "grass roots" sort which set him in motion.

The sixty-three-year-old Capell has had a long history of Radical Rightist activity—mostly as a writer and lecturer. He has written many articles for Willis Carto's right-wing *American Mercury* and has been a frequent speaker at Carto's Liberty Lobby conventions.[20] Capell's activities have also intertwined with those of the John Birch Society. He has written articles regularly for the two Birch monthlies, *American Opinion* and *Review of the News,* and has appeared at the Society's "God, Family and Country" rallies.

For the past fifteen years Capell has published his own news-letter called the *Herald of Freedom,* which has a circulation of about 5,000.[21] It was this particular newsletter which struck the first discordant note of the Radical Right's imminent cacophony on the theme of sex education.

CAPELL FIRES THE FIRST RADICAL RIGHTIST BLAST. The cacophony began when the June 14, 1968, edition of the *Herald of Freedom* published Capell's article entitled "A Look At Sex Education." In this article Capell referred to the "grass roots" opposition as what had directed his attention to sex education as an issue.

He had become aware of it through a story in the *Tustin News* of Tustin, California.[22] It described how the Tustin Elementary District Coordinating Council, an organization made up of presidents of the district's various P.T.A.s, had become aware that some of the members of the Sex Information and Education Council of the United States (SIECUS) were also involved, in one way or another, with *Sexology* magazine—a periodical that they viewed with very serious reservations on the grounds that it allegedly "exploited" human sexuality. Their concern was heightened by the fact that SIECUS had been making indirect assistance available to schools that wished to establish sex education programs.

SIECUS AND SEX EDUCATION AS A COMMUNIST PLOT.   Capell took up where the *Tustin News* left off. He charged that SIECUS mixed "innocent do-gooders with not-so-innocent plotters."[23] He then suggested who the plotters might be. He quoted "informants" who described Dr. Mary Calderone, the Executive Director of SIECUS, and her husband, Dr. Frank A. Calderone, as "ultra-liberal one-worlders."[24] Then he classified Dr. Isadore Rubin, SIECUS's treasurer, as an "identified. . .member of the Communist Party"— primarily on the basis of Rubin's alleged affiliation with the Communist Party U.S.A. during the 1940s, which was supposedly revealed in a public meeting of the House Committee on Un-American Activities in 1955.[25] (Rubin was one of those who refused to testify about his political affiliations on the grounds that the Committee had no constitutional right to compel him to do so.) Capell then quoted "information from the files of the Committee on Un-American Activities—U.S. House of Representatives" to link SIECUS' cofounder, the Rev. William H. Genne, with three "Communist fronts."[26] Finally, Capell completed his ring of "guilt by association" by pointing out that SIECUS used materials prepared by Dr. Albert Ellis, a figure charged by Capell with being a condoner of "perversion, adultery, teen-age sex and premarital sex."[27]

Capell closed his article with the following remarks.

Through the promotion of pornography, drug use and the "New Morality," the will to resist the International Communist

Conspiracy is being weakened . . . "situation ethics" and the idea
that there is no longer any "right" or "wrong" way to act, along
with downgrading of the influence of the family and religion play
right into the hands of the Communists.[28]

In retrospect, it is clear that Capell's article contained most of
the basic themes of the Radical Right's impending large-scale
attack on sex education. What followed was, in the main, a series
of variations. However, since the majority of Radical Rightist endeavors are variations on the basic themes which are detailed in
our analysis of their ideology, Capell's most basic contribution
was in calling the Right's attention to this extremely promising
auxiliary cause.

CAPELL'S ALLEGED CLAIM OF PRIMACY.   Capell, himself, claims
that his efforts were far more significant than merely calling the
Radical Right's attention to the issue. At the Birch Society's eighth
annual God, Family, and Country Rally in 1970, Capell reportedly
told visitors to his booth that *he* had done the research that led
to the Drake-directed "Christian Crusade" against SIECUS and sex
education.[29] Assuming that Capell made this claim, and there is
good reason to believe that he did, it may have been "sour grapes"
from the man who had hit "pay dirt" only to have it mined by
Hargis and company. On the other hand, if Capell's claim is true, it
must count as a vivid demonstration of the interaction and cooperation that obtains between the Fundradists and their secular counterparts.

The intensity of the campaign mounts: "Christian
Crusade" joins the attack

The opening salvo of the Fundradist's attack on sex education
was fired by Dr. Gordon Drake on Monday, June 24, 1968, over
the "Christian Crusade" radio network. A description of this first
broadcast reveals the thrust of the attack. Drake began by saying,
"I have four broadcasts here. I am primarily concerned with Sex
Education in the elementary schools, which is tied in with Sensitivity Training."[30] He then linked SIECUS to the National Educa-

tion Asociation by noting that SIECUS's executive director, Dr. Mary Calderone, had contributed to the NEA *Journal* and that NEA President-elect Elizabeth Koontz was on the board of directors of SIECUS. He then lashed out at a set of colored slides "largely designed by Dr. Mary Calderone entitled "How Babies are Made."[31]

Drake claimed the slides presented ". . .an animalistic view of sex which is shocking and completely inappropriate for children five through twelve years of age, though this is the age group they are designed for."[32]

He noted that the slides could be purchased with federal funds, exclaiming, "This is your federal tax money, mind you, which is now helping to pay for the most abominable program in the public schools."[33]

When one considers that a long-standing Fundradist demand has involved the abolition of the income tax and the elimination of federal assistance for nearly everything but "commie" hunting, this ideological stone must surely have catapulted to many a mark.

EVIDENCE THAT PUBLIC INTEREST WAS ALREADY AROUSED. Then Drake called his audience's attention to an article in that month's issue of the *Reader's Digest* entitled "Sex Education—Blunt Answers for Tough Questions." The article was based on an interview with Dr. Lester Kirkendall, a cofounder and board member of SIECUS. Drake promised that a later broadcast would furnish information that would reveal ". . .what kind of man this [Kirkendall] is."[34]

Drake's reference demonstrates that public interest in sex education had already become sufficient to warrant a feature article in *Reader's Digest*. Thus the Radical Right's discovery of this issue was probably inevitable—with or without the help of Frank Capell.

Next, Drake circuitously implicated parochial schooling by quoting bits and pieces of remarks made by the Reverend Daniel Brent, Associate Superintendent of the Rochester, New York, Catholic Schools. Even out of context, Father Brent's remarks were mild and Rochester was hardly the Vatican. But it was now clear that Drake's attack would include parochial schooling.[35]

Drake closed his first anti-sex education broadcast by quoting an alleged statement by the San Luis Obispo, California, Superintendent of Schools to the effect that "The SIECUS slides were too simple for fifth grade" and that his schools had "secured more sophisticated material."[36] Then, without offering any proof of connection, Drake listed some of SIECUS's "more sophisticated material" dealing with masturbation, homosexuality, premarital sex, and similar subjects.

The basic thrust of the Radical Rightist's attack

Although Drake had three more introductory broadcasts to go, and the rest of the Fundradists and the secular Radical Right had yet to join in the fray, the basic thrust that was to characterize the whole Radical Rightist attack on sex education was already apparent. Essentially, the theme was that sex education was the quasi-pornographic product of the insidious red-tainted organization known as SIECUS and its collaborators and dupes in the NEA, teacher training institutions, and other "liberal" establishments such as the U.S. Office of Education and the National Council of Churches. Additionally, sex education was depicted as the principal vehicle for a still larger attack on traditional Christian values, the institution of the family and, ultimately, American culture itself. Then, once these were undermined, the way would be paved for the inevitable Communist takeover.[37]

THE HONORABLE JOHN RARICK OF LOUISIANA. On the same day that Drake made his second anti–sex education broadcast (Tuesday, June 25, 1968) Congressman John R. Rarick (D.-La.) rose from his seat in Congress and observed to those present that ". . . 'filthy books' have been promoted from the corner drugstore to be made respectable by being called 'education' for our kids." Rep. Rarick linked these "filthy books" to compulsory sex education and suggested that introduction of the latter into the schools was contributing to "moral degeneracy, sex crimes and illegitimacy . . ."[38] Then Rep. Rarick had Frank Capell's previously discussed *Herald of Freedom* article "A Look at Sex Education" read into *The Congressional Record*.

Rep. Rarick has a long and extensive history of involvement with various portions of the Radical Right. For example, Rep. Rarick was one of the principal speakers at Carl McIntire's "Win the War" rally in Washington on April 5, 1970. The previous day he had personally addressed the West Coast Conference of Willis Carto's Radical Rightist "Liberty Lobby," a conference the primary purpose of which was to generate support for McIntire's rally.[39] Rep. Rarick's association with Liberty Lobby has also included his use of the official House letterhead to raise funds for their purposes.[40] Additionally, he has long been a member of the overtly racist [White] Citizens Councils.[41]

This documentation by no means exhausts the list of Rep. Rarick's activities and affiliations. And this is hardly the time or place to do so. But, in general, it is safe to conclude that the Radical Right has few stauncher advocates in Congress.[42]

Drake's innovations

In his first anti–sex education broadcast Drake had followed Capell in aligning his sights on SIECUS and its allegedly pornographic, anti-Christian, and anti-American learnings as the "bull's-eye" of the sex education target. But Drake went Capell one better when he also used this broadcast to tie the issue of sensitivity training to the controversy's tail. This was a brand-new association that, however unrelated in actual fact, was to become a major feature of the whole campaign.

As the sex education controversy grew more and more widespread, there were literally thousands of permutations and combinations of the themes struck by Drake in his very first anti–sex education broadcast. But what was remarkable about the controversy was that it rarely strayed beyond these themes.

Obviously neither Capell, Drake, the "Christian Crusade," nor the entire Radical Right could be completely responsible for this startling uniformity. But it is equally obvious that when the Radical Right discovered the sex education issue they also discovered a nerve that was capable of sending twinges of discomfort throughout the nation. And they didn't hesitate to dig at it.

THE ANTI–SEX EDUCATION BROADCASTS CONTINUE. Parts two, three, and four of Drake's four-part series against sex education were primarily elaborations of the basic themes sounded in the first broadcast. But they were also closely tied to his earlier, previously described attacks on the NEA, progressivism, UNESCO, the U.S. Office of Education, and other "liberal leftist" organizations and movements. This was Drake's own personal contribution. Of course they also included further denunciations of SIECUS and its individual board members—who were frequently attacked by name.

By the end of the final broadcast what had begun as a *relatively* bland, if simple-minded, analysis of the sex education movement had turned into a distorted diatribe which came out like this:

> The efforts of the NEA to destroy the traditional moral fiber of America and replace it with a pervasive sickly humanism is a cleverly contrived plan. Pompous authorities such as Dr. Kirkendall and Dr. Calderone deliberately spew their poison of obsessive sexuality and faceless "groupitis" [which, actually, is the Sensitivity Training goal] before the innocent and the gullible. This ideologic [sic] pablum is all too frequently swallowed by feather-headed professors, wide-eyed students, and trusting citizens out of sheer frustration. Christian morality is assessed as an ancient oddity to be studied in the same lecture as the religious supersitions of the Hottentots and the Australian Aborigines.
>
> Patriotism, too, is evil since it creates a strong feeling of competition and may even incite the citizens of a country to fight for their country, which according to Dr. Kirkendall, is immoral. The new morality is injected into most NEA projects.
>
> The strength of the NEA is in its membership. At this point we have no alternative but to rally the forces of America which still hold dear to [sic] our traditional values under God, of country and home.
>
> . . .If we do not join hands and throw out the intruders another few years will be too late.[43]

A BACKWARD GLANCE. Considering Frank Capell's alleged claim that he did Drake's research on sex education, one might wonder if his hand is visible in any of these broadcasts. The answer to that is a conditional yes.

In the first place, Drake's emphasis on SIECUS as the arch-villain does constitute a recapitulation of the major thrust of Capell's pioneering *Herald of Freedom* article. But it could be argued that this was either a coincidence or some curious variation of the "great minds run in the same channel" phenomenon.

There is, however, another piece of evidence in Drake's series of broadcasts on sex education that either reveals Capell's covert influence or constitutes a rather remarkable coincidence. On the same day that Congressman Rarick was reading Capell's article into *The Congressional Record,* Drake made his second broadcast. Near its end Drake noted that four SIECUS members were also on the Board of Consultants of *Sexology* magazine—classified by Drake as "high class smut."[44] Then, after describing the nature of an article in the June 1968 issue, Drake said,

> Other articles that have appeared in *Sexology* include "Alcohol Can Solve Sex Problems," "Group Sex Orgies," "My Wife Knows I'm Homosexual," "Gangs That Hunt Down 'Queers,'" and "Do Sex-Change Men Want to be Mothers"—written by a SIECUS board member.[45]

It will be recalled that in Capell's *Herald of Freedom* article he cited a warning regarding SIECUS from Mrs. Arthur Vandenberg of the Tustin, California, Elementary District Coordinating Council:

> Mrs. Vandenberg pointed to the fact that two editors of the *Sexology* magazine [sic] as well as two members of the "board of consultants" are also members of the SIECUS board of directors. . .
>
> Mrs. Vandenberg listed such prurient titles of articles appearing in *Sexology* as: "Alcohol can Solve Sex Problems," "Group Sex Orgies," "My wife Knows I'm Homosexual," and "Gangs That Hunt Down Queers,". . .[46]

Clearly, Drake's account of the relationships between SIECUS and *Sexology* is essentially the same as Capell's. But even more remarkably, of all the article titles available from past issues of *Sexology,* Drake cited the *same articles* as those cited by Mrs. Vandenberg *and* in the *same order*—the only novelty being that Drake added one that was not mentioned by Capell.

Of course, radio broadcasts do not lend themselves to the acknowledgment of all of one's sources. But on pages 134 and 135 of Drake's book, *Blackboard Power: NEA Threat to America,*[47] marketed soon after his anti-sex education broadcast series, Drake listed the *same articles* in the *same order,* only this time he credited the April 30, 1968, issue of the right-wing Anaheim, California, *Bulletin.*[48] Curiously, the reference department of the Anaheim Public Library was unable to locate any such reference in the *Bulletin* on either that date or April 3, 1968 (the latter checked on the assumption that there might have been a printing error).[49]

This confusion of origins is further complicated by Drake's pamphlet entitled, *Is The School House the Proper Place to Teach Raw Sex?*[50] This pamphlet was published shortly after Drake's book and became "one of the most widely distributed pieces of propaganda"[51] to appear during the controversy. In it Drake cited a *Sexology* article on "The Prostitutes of Ancient Greece," a title not mentioned in Capell's article, and credits it to the April 25, 1968, edition of the *Tustin News.*[52] (Interestingly, it was this particular edition and, in fact, this same article that was Capell's primary source.) Then, compounding the problem, Drake listed those *same titles* in that *same order* again. But this time he gave no credit at all.[53]

Summing up the origins of the controversy

Our backward glance at Capell's alleged claim that he did the research for Drake and Hargis' "Christian Crusade" against sex education suggests that either Drake's documentation and acknowledgements regarding this particular matter were extremely lax or he was sidestepping the matter of their actual origin. But, based on Drake's eight-part series of broadcasts against the NEA in March of that year, it is clear that he and Hargis had already decided to attack the state of public education and develop it as an auxiliary cause. It seems likely that when the issue of sex education presented itself Drake simply plugged it into his NEA conspiracy theme and added the "sensitivity training" touch. So, in that sense, even if Drake did use Capell's "plug," it is unlikely that is all he did. But we are still left with the very real possibility that we have uncovered an unsurprising but interesting case of covert collaboration between the secular and Fundradist wings of the Radical Right.

The fact of identical dates for Rep. Rarick's Congressional speech and Drake's second broadcast (both sharing similar themes, citing the *same Sexology references* in the *same order* and probably sharing the same primary source) suggests the possibility of another case of collaboration. In this case it would be collaboration between the extremist fringe and a member of Congress to strike the same nerve at the same time.

Some cautionary remarks

The Radical Right was involved in the generation of the controversy over sex education virtually from its beginning. What is more, it was Billy James Hargis' "Christian Crusade," with the special assistance of Dr. Gordon Drake, which did more than any other organization to push the matter to public prominence and simultaneously move it from the level of basic but civil disagreement to that of unreasoning hysteria.

But in order to keep this appraisal in proper perspective several qualifying remarks are in order. First, as was mentioned previously, by early 1968 the sex education movement was well along and grass roots opposition to it, not all of it Radical Rightist by any means, was already developing *before* Hargis and company jumped aboard. After all, sex is a central American anxiety and any attempt to deal with it in our schools must inevitably generate controversy. So, in that sense at least, the Fundradists and other Radical Rightists did not *create* the controversy so much as they *exploited* it.

This, in turn, calls for acknowledging that much public concern about sex education was, and is, multifaceted, deep and quite reasonable. It is clearly *not* the case that opposition to certain varieties of sex education is symptomatic of either Radical Rightist tendencies or wrong-headedness. The first portion of the analysis in this chapter concentrates on the Radical Right and its Fundradist element because that is our center of interest and *not* because we presume them to be the sole cause of the controversy.

Even considering these cautions, however, several facts continue to stand out. First, the Radical Right, and most especially its Fundradist element, *did* play an extremely important, even pivotal role in the generation and continuation of the controversy. Second, and more importantly, it was the unreasonable, unappeasable, and frequently irresponsible nature of their opposition which, more than any other single factor, helped to polarize public opinion, eliminate the middle ground, and make responsible dialogue extremely difficult, if not impossible.

Rarely, if ever, did the Fundradists and their secular brethren responsibly confront the proponents of sex education with the many hard and painful questions that needed to be raised. Instead, they "sounded trail" every time the scent of fear or mistrust wafted their way. And it wasn't long before they had groups of citizens running in "full cry" after their own fantasies, all but drowning out the voices of those who wished to discuss alternatives.

The fact that a sexual issue could be used with such devastating effectiveness by the various components of the Radical Right is, in itself, evidence of the dismal state of the nation's sexual adjustment and the concomitant need for some sort of education in these matters.[54]

What kind of education this should be requires very careful consideration. But that is precisely the kind of consideration that the Fundradists and the rest of the Radical Right rendered virtually impossible through the nature of their opposition.

3

The gathering storm

Throughout the summer of 1968 Drake and Hargis continued to develop public antipathy toward the general state of education as an auxiliary cause. But as the summer wore on, it became increasingly clear that the "Christian Crusade" was beginning to regard sex education as the issue with the most potential.

Blackboard power: NEA threat to America

In August of 1968 Drake's book *Blackboard Power: NEA Threat to America* was finally published after nearly six months of promotion. Much of the book mirrored the themes struck by Drake in his first series of "Crusade" broadcasts in March. For example, it contained the new standard attacks on the NEA's cooperation with UNESCO, the World Confederation of Organizations of the Teaching Profession, and the U.S. Office of Education;[1] the growing militancy of teachers which had led to their increasing use of sanctions or strikes;[2] and on "Progressivism," John Dewey, George S. Counts, Harold Rugg, and other promoters of "the New Education."[3]

Chapter 10 was a spin-off from the issues of sex education

and sensitivity training, which had been the themes of Drake's June broadcasts. In fact, much of the wording was the same as that used in the broadcasts. The major target was again SIECUS and its "lefty liberal" collaborators in the educational community.

The significance of the inclusion of this chapter in Drake's book is *not* simply its similarity to his earlier broadcasts or to the material of Frank Capell—though both of these facts are noteworthy. Exhibiting timing suggestive of a definite purpose, it was published less than one month before school began and closed with instructions concerning "What Can Parents Do?" to ". . .protect their children from immoral instruction in the public schools. . . ."[4]

Tactics

Drake urged parents to work within their circle of friends and in their churches and clubs; to contact the local newspaper and write letters to the editor; and to write or personally contact local and state representatives as well as teachers, administrators, and school boards.

He suggested forming "ad hoc groups" such as MOMS (Mothers Organized for Moral Stability; POSE (Parents Opposed to Sex Education); or SOS (Save Our Schools)—all of which were in existence when Drake made his June broadcasts. He advocated calling radio talk shows and "using the information in this book," as well as "putting out mimeographed broadsides of your own."[5] He also suggested organizing meetings and obtaining a speaker who could "speak, debate and analyze with professional assistance the precise curriculum being used in your schools."[6]

Then, providing an example of the "this is the argument upon which I base my facts" reasoning which came to be characteristic of the "anti" campaign, Drake admonished parents to

> Determine its [the sex education program's] lack of moral orientation and defiance of a practical law of learning which dictates materials be presented to students at their point of maturation and need.[7]

Finally, reflecting several of the Fundradist characteristics described in the ideological and theoretical analysis that comes later,
Drake suggested that parents should *"Expose* and *depose* through
school board pressures those teachers and administrators who do
not reflect your community's mores" and "Ask the local newspaper to editorialize—*if the editor supports your point of view."*[8]
(Emphasis mine.) Of course, all of these instructions came after
a sensational description of sex education as an anti-Christian, un-
American, Communist plot that had been birthed from the bowels
of Hell.

Many of the tactics which Drake advocated in this chapter
would be sensible procedures for organizing public opposition on
many different issues. So, in this respect, it is hardly remarkable
that when the controversy grew to truly massive proportions it was
characterized by precisely these methods. What *is remarkable* and
distressing is that, in the main, the opposition not only organized
in the fashion suggested by Drake, but frequently invited him
to be the speaker and used his allegations in making charges in
their own community.

Rarely was the actual content of the local program, if there
even was one, subjected to any scrutiny. Instead, it was the allegations of Drake and company that kept getting the play. Over and
over again the issues revolved around the charge that SIECUS
was the major command post for a conspiracy to subvert America
by corrupting the morals of its youth and cutting the bonds that
hold the nuclear family together. This would be accomplished
through the destruction of "Christian morality" and the introduction of sexual license, perversion, pornography, and ultimately
an epidemic of unwanted pregnancies and venereal disease. The
conspiracy thesis has always been a central feature of the Fundradists' ideology. And it was the heart of their attack on sex education.

THE EXAMPLE OF WESTFIELD, NEW JERSEY. By way of example,
the community of Westfield, New Jersey, suspended its "Family
Living Program" after a bitter controversy that was described in

a television documentary as "tearing the town apart." In commenting on the controversy one of the local medical doctors, who favored the program, said "Every issue seemed to go back to SIECUS."[9] This *despite* the fact that "very little, *if any*, SIECUS materials were even involved."[10]

As a matter of fact, according to a SIECUS spokesman that organization has *never* been involved in providing materials for students.[11] Its efforts have been directed toward providing materials for teachers—a point that Drake continually failed to acknowledge and that others usually overlooked. Yet, time and again, the Fundradists' charges of conspiracy centered on SIECUS as the instrument of Communist subversion.

Is the Schoolhouse the Proper Place to Teach Raw Sex?

It has already been noted that Drake's pamphlet *Is the Schoolhouse the Proper Place to Teach Raw Sex?** was one of the most widely distributed pieces of propaganda[12] to appear during the controversy. The pamphlet was published in September of 1968 —one month after *Blackboard Power* was released and the same month that most schools opened.

The pamphlet was primarily an elaboration of Drake's earlier broadcasts and the allegations in chapter 10 of his book. However, its forty-page size, fifty-cent price, and sensational rhetorical title made it a very effective instrument for the dissemination of the "Christian Crusade's" views.

Drake's charges against SIECUS, sex education, and sensitivity training have already been outlined in some detail. But because of its wide circulation and the fact that it is particularly revealing of Drake's methods, this pamphlet merits a brief appraisal.

As its beginning Drake quotes a speech by Dr. Mary Calderone, SIECUS's director, that was allegedly made to a group of boys at Blair Academy in New Jersey. Drake quotes Dr. Calderone as

---

*Drake spells "schoolhouse" both as one word and as two. For instance, it is two on the outside cover of his pamphlet but one word on the title page. I tried to mirror his confused usage throughout this section.   —Author

saying "What is sex for? It's for fun. . .for wonderful sensation. . .
. Sex is not something you turn off like a faucet. If you do, it's un-
healthy."[13] *In context* Dr. Calderone's actual remarks were:

> What is sex for? It's for fun, that I know, for wonderful sen-
> sations. It's also for reproduction, sedation, rewards, punishment.
> It's a status symbol, a commercial come-on, proof of indepen-
> dence, a form of emotional blackmail. Many of these are nega-
> tive ways of using sex. What we are trying to feel our way
> toward is positive ways. Sex is not something to be feared or
> degraded or kicked around or used. Sex is not something you
> turn off like a faucet. If you do, it's unhealthy. We are sexual
> beings, legitimately so, at every age. Don't think that sex stops
> at 50. We need new values to establish when and how we should
> have sexual experiences.[14]

The reader can decide Drake's purpose in omitting what he
did from the context of Dr. Calderone's remarks.

Drake also told of how Dr. Calderone told the Blair Academy
students ". . .I don't believe. . .the old 'Thou shalt nots' apply anymore."[15] She actually said, "I am a religious person, but I don't
believe the old thou-shalt-nots apply anymore." And she said it to
the National Conference of Parents and Teachers, *not* to the students of Blair Academy. Finally, Drake derived *both* of these
quotes from a *Look* magazine article entitled "Sex Education
Comes of Age,"[16] which made it perfectly clear that Dr. Calderone
was attempting to *describe* the conditions of American society, not
sanction them.[17]

All of these errors and omissions occur on the very first content
page of Drake's pamphlet. So, whatever can be said for Dr. Drake's
motives, it is clear that his research was off to an inauspicious beginning.

Of course, the pamphlet contains Drake's curiously repetitive list
of "randomly" selected articles from *Sexology* magazine that we
have already discussed. But it is also replete with statements like
the following.

> **Reverends Fletcher and Genne and Drs. Kirkendall, Cal-
> derone, Rubin and Ellis leave little to the imagination in their**

stand against Biblical morality, and in their *purpose of promoting
free sex* in the schools of America.[18] [Emphasis mine]

Reviewing a selection of these individuals' writings reveals that
they do indeed advocate the abolition of the kind of "Biblical
moralty" that helped Hawthorne's Hester win her *A*. But they most
certainly do *not* advocate complete sexual license, as Drake's term
"free sex" suggests. On the contrary, their respective opinions on
human sexuality generally reveal a profound desire to enrich and
strengthen sexual morality rather than destroy it.[19]

In one curious passage Drake describes the "unbelievably clever
models" of "plastic human figures with interchangeable male and
female sex organs," which are used for instructional purposes in
some schools as "instant transvestism."[20]

There are also lurid and *undocumented* tales describing classroom demonstrations of the "application of a condrum [sic] on a
life-size plastic phallus"[21] and the installation of "desensitizing joint
boy-girl toilet facilities without partitions."[22]

Passages such as these, as well as cruder materials produced
later by local activists, suggest that, for some people at least, anti–
sex education literature serves as a form of Puritanical pornography.

Drake summarized these contentions of his pamphlet with the following passage.

> It should be evident that the sex educators are in league with
> the sexologists—who represent every shade of muddy gray
> morality, ministers colored atheistic pink, and camp followers
> of every persuasion—off-beat psychiatrists to ruthless publishers
> of pornography. The enemy is formidable at first glance, but
> becomes awesomely powerful when we discover the interlocking
> directorates and working relationship of national organizations
> which provide havens for these degenerates.[23]

He then issued a program of action for local citizens, closing
with the reminder that "Charges have always been made by a
small corp [sic] of highly organized or disciplined people who
are dedicated to their cause."[24] In this case, the events of the next
two years would prove him quite right.

The grounds for success

During this initial period Drake, through Hargis' "Christian Crusade," emerged as the prime mover in the attack on sex education. Through broadcasts, his book, his pamphlet, sympathetic editorials, and word of mouth his charges spread with remarkable rapidity throughout the nation.

This was facilitated by the fact that the whole issue of sex education was being scrutinized with increasing interest by the mass media.[25] The general public was becoming more and more aware of the trend toward sex education programs in the nation's schools. And while most citizens approved of such courses, many other reacted in an actively negative fashion.[26]

Peripheral groups opposed to sex education had begun to form even before Drake or Capell had latched on to the issues. But Drake's "Crusade," with its sensational charges and dichotomous answers, motivated many local Fundradists, or their secular counterparts, to organize committees and begin fighting what they perceived to be a threat to their children. These groups provided a focal point for reaction. And they soon began to attract individuals who *were not* on the political fringe but *were* terribly disturbed over sex education or, at least, over what they *thought* it to be.

Of course, non–Radical Rightists also formed anti–sex education committees. Sometimes these committees remained free from Rightist influence and served as constructive and responsible critics of existing or proposed programs. Unfortunately, despite these responsible beginnings, they were prone to end up as part of the Radical Rightist cause.

The pace of sex education's adoption

The coalescence of public opposition to sex education in the schools was facilitated by the fact that, although this particular curriculum innovation had proceeded at a gradual pace until 1963 or 1964, change then began to come with remarkable speed. By 1967 experts were estimating that in another two years fully seventy percent of the nation's schools would have sex education.[27]

The speed of this change intensified public reaction against it. You cannot change a society's treatment of sex from silent embarrassment to open discussion in a classroom without rubbing a lot of public hair the wrong way. And this pertains even if the discussion is really an essentially mindless perpetuation of middle-class morality with only a veneer of objectivity. Additionally, these changes were coming about at precisely the same time that the "Age of Aquarius" was in full and threatening blossom. And even though some of the demand for sex education was intensified by this flowering, so too was a good deal of its opposition.

In short, Drake and company could hardly have picked a better cause *or* time. And the success of their efforts during the 1968–69 school year stands as evidence of that fact.

Drake's impact: The example of Anaheim

The impact of Drake's "Crusade" broadcasts and publications was different in each community that it touched. Examining these variations would make a prohibitive demand on both time and space. But by teasing out Drake's initial impact on the Family Life and Sex Education (FLSE) program in the Anaheim, California, Union High School District, we can become familiar with a typical pattern of impact and simultaneously learn the basic facts regarding the most famous sex education controversy of them all.

The Anaheim Union High School District takes up forty square miles of Orange County, a political entity with a previously noted reputation for a high incidence of right-wing extremists. However unlikely such a locale may seem as a place to launch a pioneer sex education program, that is precisely what the Anaheim High School District set out in 1964 to do. (The first course actually began in the spring of 1965.[28])

This seeming anomaly is only partially explained by a 1963 poll in the District which revealed ninty percent of the adult population in favor of sex education in school.[29] Additionally, since

World War II, Anaheim has become a "bedroom suburb" of Los Angeles; as such, it has served as a fertile ground for the development of alienation, anomie, and the other symptoms of the social upheavals of the last three decades. Such a situation paradoxically creates a greater need for sex education in school while simultaneously encouraging the sort of political extremism that opposes it on a purely emotional level. These factors also aid us in understanding this seeming anomaly. Perhaps the right-wing reputation of this area is more a consequence of the local Radical Right's stridency and fervor than it is their numbers.

The Anaheim course series was designed to deal with issues that transcended human sexuality. Hence its name, "Family Life and Sex Education." It was initially conducted on the seventh-grade level, lasted four and one-half weeks, emphasized discussion, and was developed in close consultation with various groups within the community.[30]

In an effort to sidestep the impossible task of determining *whose* particular moral values would prevail if an official position on such things as premarital intercourse were to be adopted, the course ostensibly emphasized the importance of individual choice in this and similar matters. Nevertheless, the course was rich in cautionary tales regarding veneral disease and unwanted pregnancies. So much so, in fact, that one observer remarked that the course's main message was, "If you play, you'll pay."[31] What the students were encouraged to think about was simply, what they would "pay," and to whom, if they were to "mess around." "Playing" was clearly out of the question so far as the program was concerned.

Anaheim's FLSE program encountered few difficulties in its first two years. In fact, the program garnered a great deal of favorable publicity through articles in national magazines which cited it as something of a model.

But in late August of 1968[32] Mrs. Eleanor Howe, wife of a career Marine officer and mother of four, requested at an Anaheim school board meeting that she and several others be permitted to give a special presentation on the FLSE program. Her request was denied.[33]

Shortly thereafter Mrs. Howe wrote an angry letter to the board requesting that her twin sons, who were then in eleventh grade, be excused from the program on the grounds that one of them had been acutely embarrassed when the course's teacher had posed a hypothetical question as to what the Howe boy would do if he caught his son in the act of masturbating. (The boy had recommended punishment and the class apparently laughed.)

Such requests to be excused were routinely approved, so no trouble was encountered there. But Mrs. Howe also sent a copy of her letter to the right-wing Anaheim *Bulletin*.[34] Upon its publication Mrs. Howe became the focal point of an ever-increasing opposition to the program. Public pressure began to build—demanding a special meeting to be devoted to Mrs. Howe's presentation on the FLSE program. The pressure was loosely organized around a group calling themselves the Citizen's Committee for California —once the political vehicle of Senator Goldwater.[35] Superintendent Paul Cook advised against such a meeting. But the board eventually overruled him and scheduled a special "workshop" for October.[36]

When the "workshop" took place Mrs. Howe, backed by then State Senator John Schmitz, an acknowledged Birch Society member, presented an obviously well-prepared slide and tape show attacking the FLSE program.[37] The thrust of Mrs. Howe's presentation was that Anaheim's FLSE program was a creature of SIECUS and that this particular organization was the nucleus of a plot to undermine the family, God, and country.[38]

The general tone of the attack suggested that Mrs. Howe had gathered her ammunition in some right-wing powder room. And a closer inspection would later reveal that she had indeed—and without acknowledgement—lifted whole passages from Drake's *Is the School House the Proper Place to Teach Raw Sex?*[39] But at that time the "Crusade's" campaign against sex education was not common knowledge and the program's proponents were forced to defend themselves with dangerously incomplete information regarding the nature, or even the identity, of their primary antagonists.

SIECUS had *not* even been chartered until *after* the FLSE program had been launched. What is more, SIECUS had written to Anaheim in order to gain information regarding the program fully two years after its inception.[40] But from the time of that "workshop" the anti-FLSE forces attended one school board meeting after another, loudly voicing their disquiet regarding sex, SIECUS, and subversion.

The Anaheim *Bulletin* did its part by publishing "exposés" of the program and / or SIECUS and by eventually featuring an anti-sex education column by John Steinbacher who later gained dubious notoriety as the producer of a record album called *The Child Seducers.*[41]

Ultimately, the Anaheim controversy became a center of national attention. Some of the very same publications which had cited Anaheim's FLSE as a pioneer and model were now pointing to the struggle surrounding it as the microcosm of a national battle.[42]

Both the program and Superintendent Paul Cook were ultimately ousted from Anaheim following a crucial school board election in which only fourteen percent of the electorate voted. Why there was such a small turnout for an election that had bceome a matter of national interest was something of a puzzle. Ex-Superintendent Cook speculated that it was a combination of apathy bred of alienation and a related feeling of powerlessness, plus a dose of good, old-fashioned fear.[43]

But whatever the explanation for the low turnout, there could be little doubt that no one had a right to stand more triumphantly in the wreckage than Dr. Gordon V. Drake and the "Christian Crusade."

4

Deluge

During the 1968–69 school year, the controversy over school-based sex education grew from a murmur to an uproar that began to rival the evolution controversy that gripped American education during the 1920s. In fact, the controversy grew so quickly that some officials of the NEA described it as a "sex-plosion."[1]

SIECUS began to see evidence that something was afoot shortly after Capell, Congressman Rarick, and Drake attempted to link that organization and the sex education movement with subversion, moral degeneracy, and anti-Americanism. For instance, just one month after the attacks began SIECUS received several letters posted in New Orleans, Louisiana (Rep. Rarick's home state), which were addressed as follows:

> (A disgrace to the *holy* name)[2]
> Mary Stincken Calderone, tool of Satan & the Zionists
> SIECUS rats of Moscow
> Rat nest—1855 Broadway
> N.Y. NY [sic]

45

> Sex-seducers & Sex-Maniacs
> Christenden, Gendel, Macy, Rigler & Lief
> Parasites, Puppets & Prostitutes
> of
> Communist Isador Rubin
> Mary *STINKEN* Calderone, *M*istress of the *D*evil;
>   *M*isfit *P*rostitute of *H*ell
> 1855 Broadway
> NY NY [sic]

> Female Rat Mary Stienken Calderone, Isador Rubin (Comm.
>   Rat) & Sex Perverts, [sic] Sexologists & Red Rat Finks of
>   *S*ex-maniacs *I*n seducing *E*very *C*hild *U*nder *S*atans [sic]
>   directives
> 1835 Broadway
> NY.
> NY. [sic]

The body of the last letter reads as follows:

> Read Matt. 23:15 & Quake & Shudder!
> God said, about seducers of children: about *you*" you will wish
> you had never been born. . .and:
>   you'd be *Better off* if a millstone were tied around your
>   neck, & you be cast into the *depths* of the sea. [sic]
>   He meant that the drowning would be better than being
>   cast into the depths of *Hell* where you will have *molten*
>   steel *poured* into you from both directions. . .& where your
>   diet will be puss, excretions, roaches, maggots & spiders.
>   Think it over in bed *tonite*, as well as on your death bed.
>   [sic]
>
> *Unsigned*[3]

Initially, this "first of the hate mail" could be looked upon as
nothing more than the product of a single twisted mind. But
as the controversy developed, these early letters came to sym-
bolize an all-too-common characteristic of the controversy. Nearly
everywhere that it spread throughout the nation, the sadly vulgar
utterances of those on or beyond the edge of reason were mani-
fested in anonymous telephone calls, hate mail, unsigned literature,
and ugly threats. And many of them reflected the sensational distortions of the Radical Right, just as these first letters did.

Drake takes to the road

September 1968 marked both the release of Drake's *Is the School-house the Proper Place to Teach Raw Sex?* and the "Christian Crusade" launching of a speaking tour which eventually covered the country. The topic was sex education and the featured speaker was usually Gordon Drake. During most of the 1968–69 school year, Drake spent an average of three out of every four weeks on the road. He crisscrossed the country delivering the "Gospel" about SIECUS, sex and subversion, encouraging "anti" groups to organize, and selling the "Crusade's" publications.[4]

Sometimes he was joined by Charles Secrest and David Noebel, both on the "Crusade" staff, and they would form a "Family, Schools and Morality" seminar team that conducted two-day sessions. One such "seminar" was held in Arlington, Virginia, on February 20 and 21, 1969. It began with Drake's basic talk on sex education with suitable alterations for that locale. Drake was followed by Charles Secrest, who took up where Drake left off— tying sex education in ". . .with the churches and what is taking place in America today in relationship to youth, sex, church and the basket of socialism."[5] The next day David Noebel took the podium to expose "rhythmic activities [and] hypnotic type music. A discussion on the subversion of young people from the cradle [sic]." He also spoke on ". . .the Communist subversion of American fold music" and ". . .Rock and Roll; primarily a discussion of the Beatles."[6] Both of Noebel's talks were obviously based on his "Christian Crusade" publications, *Rhythm, Riots and Revolution* and *Communism Hypnotism and the Beatles.*[7]

At other times Noebel and Secrest conducted independent speaking tours while Drake was busy elsewhere. For example, from April 4 through 9, 1970, the two were in Rochester and Minneapolis, Minnesota, and Des Moines, Mason City, Chariton, and Batavia, Iowa. And, just like Dr. Drake, everywhere they went they distributed literature and attempted to fortify existing groups of "antis" or to simulate the growth of new ones.

The harvest begins

The NEA had been aware of the Radical Right's attacks virtually from the beginning. They were aware, for example, long before the event, that Drake's *Blackboard Power* was going to be published.[8] But the NEA's first tangible evidence that the "Crusade's" campaign was actually bearing fruit came with the arrival of requests from affiliated locals for assistance in coping with the attack.

Some examples of this type of request follow, but with specific identifying data deliberately omitted.[9]

One such request, dated November 1, 1968, from a state education association in the South, said,

> Would you please send us the information you have on *Blackboard Power—NEA Threat to America*. . . This particular bit of poison is causing us considerable trouble in one of our more conservative areas.

A letter from an NEA local in Utah dated November 11, 1968, demonstrated another aspect of the problem. It stated in part,

> We have had a great deal of material being sent to our teachers by Christian Crusade. The article *Is the School House the Proper Place to Teach Raw Sex?* is one which is causing a wave of concern. . . . We have had many calls from teachers relative to the part Elizabeth Koontz [the NEA president at this time] is reported to have in the SIECUS program. Several have indicated they will withdraw their NEA memberships.

Still another variation on Drake's influence can be seen in a letter from a local Indiana affiliate dated December 10, 1968. It contained the following.

> One of the Board Members of the ———— ———— School System requested that I, as President of the Local Association and affiliate of NEA, read a book and discussed [sic] its contents with him. The book by Dr. Gordon V. Drake, *Blackboard Power*, looks like a regular rightwing job on the NEA. . .
>
> I am anxious to help dissuade any fears the Board member has. If it is at all possible to provide an answer to some of Dr.

Drake's allegations, I would surely appreciate whatever you have. Our Board Member is a sincere man, though, I suspect, somewhat misguided. Because he is an influential person in our community I would surely like to do all I could in a rational manner to set his mind at ease about NEA.

The opposition broadens

With the relatively inconsequential exception of Frank Capell, the early leadership of the anti–sex education campaign was drawn from the Christian Crusade. But as the popularity of the cause became increasingly apparent the remainder of the Radical Right began to get involved.

One of the first secular Radical Rightist organizations to join the campaign was "Let Freedom Ring." This particular child of the Right was delivered from our body politic by William G. Douglass, M.D., of Sarasota, Florida. By dialing an unlisted telephone number in most of the larger cities of the nation the caller can hear a ninety-second "patriotic message" that changes once a week.[10] For one such week in December 1968, "Let Freedom Ring" asked "Is the schoolhouse the proper place to teach raw sex?" This opener was followed by a ninety-second commentary on sex, SIECUS and subversion which suggested that the caller might have gotten "Crusade" headquarters by mistake.[11]

But it was not until January 1969, fully nine months after the Christian Crusade opened its campaign, that the John Birch Society officially denounced sex education. In the January 1969 *John Birch Society Bulletin,* a monthly newsletter which supplements *American Opinion,* Robert Welch announced discovery of an ". . .evil and extensive plot. . ." which involved a ". . .Communist plan to destroy the moral character of a generation."[12]

Just as Capell, Drake, and Rarick did before him, Welch laid this "plot" at the feet of SIECUS and their collaborators and dupes in the liberal educational establishment. Precisely how or why Welch decided to commit the Birch Society to the anti–sex education campaign is not clear—though it seems almost certain to have had something to do with the Christian Crusade's success with the issue.

In any event, Welch was certainly aware of and indebted to the efforts of Dr. Drake. In this, his first written pronouncement on sex education, Welch said, ". . .the best concise survey of the whole development [of the "plot" to subvert American youth through sex education] that we have seen is a pamphlet, *Is the Schoolhouse the Proper Place to Teach Raw Sex?*"[13] Soon this pamphlet was being sold in the Society's American Opinion bookstores across the country.

In this same article, Welch announced that the Birch Society was launching a "movement to restore decency." This was the genesis of the notorious MOTOREDE committees. These groups operate as "fronts" for the society and eventually attracted the support of thousands of citizens who would otherwise have rejected any such association.[14] Soon MOTOREDE committees became an integral part of hundreds of local struggles and contributed a good deal to the confusion and acrimony which characterized the controversy.

In the February 1969 *Bulletin,* Welch reiterated the charges initially made in the January issue. But he also noted that the Society was prepared to disseminate the addresses of local committees and that it invited "the participation of good citizens everywhere."[15]

In March 1969 the Society's *American Opinion* magazine, a publication with a much wider circulation than the *Bulletin,* featured a lead article entitled "Sex Education Problems" by Gary Allen.[16] Like the Radical Rightist attacks that preceded it, Allen's attack centered on SIECUS and branched out in predictable directions. In fact, the article was strikingly similar to Drake's . . . *Raw Sex. . .* pamphlet. For example, on pages 5 and 6 of Allen's article (reprinted) we find that this "top authority on civil turmoil and the New Left," made *precisely* the *same* errors and omissions in quoting Dr. Mary Calderone that Gordon Drake had made on page 2 of *Is the Schoolhouse the Proper Place to Teach Raw Sex?*[17] Yet, strangely enough, Allen made no mention of Drake in any manner whatsoever.

The John Birch Society is the largest Radical Rightist group in America. When they joined the anti–sex education campaign in early 1969 results were considerable. All of the resources of a five-million-dollar-a-year organization were now at the service of the cause. What is more, all of those dozens of relatively minor organizations which carry on a symbiotic existence within the shadow of the Birch Society were now encouraged to begin feeding on the bits and pieces thrown off from the center of the struggle.

Many Birchers had already begun their own "anti" activities within the general framework established by the Christian Crusade, and the official addition of these quasi-respectable, main-street reactionaries in secular stripe did much to legitimize and urbanize the rustic cries of doom being sounded by Hargis' Fundradists. This in turn tended to increase the number of individuals who joined the anti–sex education campaign as a result of their own anxieties regarding human sexuality and their ignorance regarding the true nature of what they were joining.[18]

The "front" device was actually so effective that many individuals refused to believe that MOTOREDE was not the independent movement that it purported to be. But, any doubt that MOTOREDE was the creation of the Birch Society could have been dispelled by examining the affiliations of its twelve-man board. Seven of the twelve, including the chairman, were members of the Birch Society's policy Council. Three others were regular contributors to Birch publications and the eleventh member, Lt. Governor Lester Maddox of Georgia, annually proclaimed a John Birch Society Day when he was Governor.[19] And while MOTOR-EDE is rather moribund at the moment, there is no evidence that its nature or origins have changed.

Soon after the Birch Society's entrance into the controversy there occurred a very noticeable shift in the activities of other Radical Rightist groups in the same direction. Organization after organization began disseminating its own variations on the theme of sex, SIECUS, and subversion until literally hundreds of bewilderingly intertwined groups were contributing to the cacophony.

Dan Smoot of the *Dan Smoot Report* and Willis Carto's *Liberty Lobby* were typical of the larger secular Radical Rightist activists and organizations who took up the cudgel. Smoot, an ex-

FBI agent who specializes in the identification of "subversives," contributed his monthly newsletter and broadcasting network (then totaling sixty-five radio and twenty-five TV stations) to the anti campaign.[20] The Liberty Lobby added financial resources commensurate with its annual estimated income of $1,000,000 but also the voice of the *Liberty Letter,* with its monthly circulation of over 250,000.[21]

Since it was a Fundamentalist group—the Christian Crusade— that brought the sex education controversy to national prominence and since restrictions on human sexuality have always been closely intertwined with Fundamentalism, it was predictable that other Fundradists would find sex education an ideal auxiliary cause. And they did.

Virtually all of the prominent Fundradists soon took up the issue as their own. Even Carl McIntire, who had lost Drake to Hargis under circumstances that encouraged enmity, found time to issue a packet containing most of the standard charges and to appear before a joint New Jersey legislative hearing on the matter.[22]

But McIntire was beset by dangerously mounting difficulties involving state accreditation of Shelton College, license renewal for Faith Seminary's radio station, WXUR, and open rebellion within the American Council of Christian Churches. Additionally, he was planning and promoting his own auxiliary cause—a demand for "victory in Vietnam" backed by a series of state and national marches. These factors tended to curb McIntire's anti– sex education efforts.

However, much of this slack was taken up by rising young activists such as Dr. William Stuart McBirnie and his "Voice of Americanism" movement. Operating out of his church in Glendale, California, McBirnie concentrated on the issue through broadcasting over some 60 stations,[23] and by publishing pamphlets such as *The Truth About the New Sex Education in the Schools* (primarily Drake's . . .*Raw Sex.* . . revisited) and *Sex and Subversion.* The latter darkly suggested that a "Homosexual International" was operating as ". . . a sort of auxiliary of the Communist International."[24] He also produced his own long-playing record album entitled *Sex Education,* which was essentially an elaboration of his first pamphlet. It did, however, contain that by now familiar passage about the interconnection between *Sexology* and *SIECUS* and the oft-repeated *Sexology* article titles first cited in the *Tustin Daily News.*[25]

And whatever vacuum remained after the "rising young activists" rushed in was quickly filled by a host of local preachers and lay persons who cranked out reams of material. Mary Breasted describes the extent of this deluge when telling of her first efforts to do background research on the controversy in Anaheim.

> It seemed that every right-wing pamphleteer, radio preacher, committee organizer, and freelance Commie-hater of indeterminate stripe had taken up the standard of all-American decency. Their numbers were staggering, and they put out information at such rapid rate that I despaired of consuming it all. Even the Anti-Defamation League, with its scores of researchers doing nothing but collecting and filing the publications of the God, Country and Motherhood types, could not fit every last pamphlet into its books on the Radical Right.[26]

The harvest continues

As opposition broadened and the resources at the disposal of the anti–sex education forces grew apace, the results of their campaign became more and more apparent:

In April of 1969, only three months after the Birch Society had joined the fight and just eight months after Drake had released his . . .*Raw Sex.* . . pamphlet, SIECUS received some 4,000 clippings, largely from small-town dailies, that contained attacks on their organization and on sex education in the public schools.[27]

The NEA continued to receive letters from beleaguered schools. One from a county superintendent in California dated April 4, 1969, read in part,

> During recent months, the public schools of our country have been under severe attack in regards to family life education and group counseling. An organization called "Families United of _____ County" has, through coercion, half-truths,

and intimidations, forced a temporary withdrawal of both of
these programs by school boards.

We obviously see the fine hand of the John Birch society
and so on down the line. . . .

The letter closed with a plea for help.

Another letter from a state education association in the far west
dated April 8 said,

> I wish to request a full and complete report concerning the
> position of the NEA in regard to sex education. ———
> among other states is becoming a hot bed of extreme right-
> wing elements who are attacking the schools on a number of
> issues. The latest "kick" is sex education, of which we have
> very little within the scope of school curriculum. . . .
>
> Specifically, I need to know what connection the NEA has
> with SIECUS? What is the function of SIECUS and who is
> involved with this organization? . . .
>
> I would appreciate hearing from you as soon as possible. I
> need the requested information immediately. . . .

A portion of a letter sent to the NEA on July 11, 1969, by the
Superintendent of Schools in a major eastern city to the NEA
completes the picture.

> I sincerely appreciated your call concerning sex education.
> We are experiencing an almost landslide opposition from false
> information disseminated by the John Birch Society and funda-
> mentalist religious groups. . . .

Another pecularity of the controversy was the proliferation of
local committees with delightful acronyms. These included
MOTOREDE, the Movement to Restore Decency; TACT, Truth
about Civil Turmoil; MOMS, Mothers for Moral Stability; PORE,
Parents opposed to Sex Education; COST, Citizens Opposing Sex
Training; PROMISE, Parents Reserve the Option of Morality in
Sex Education; POISE, Persons Opposed to Institutional Sex Edu-
cation; TASTE, Truth About Sex Training in Education; and
OOPS, the Oshkosh Organization of Parents.[28]

Precisely how many of these organizations were essentially
Radical Rightist or, more specifically, Fundradist in character is

difficult to establish. But there can be little doubt, given the nearly ubiquitous involvement of Radical Rightists in the "anti" movement, that many of these organizations were either completely or partially in that camp. This judgment is further substantiated by the unusually large numbers of local MOTOREDE, TACT, POSE, and MOMS chapters. For all of these organizations had ties with either the Birch Society or the Christian Crusade.[29]

Along with these organizations, there were a substantial number of local churches and pastors who took an active role in opposing sex education using essentially the same tactics as the Radical Right. Again, it is difficult to separate the obvious Fundradists from those who were simply committed to this particular cause. But, in any event, local church opposition played an important role in the controversy.[30]

Another product of the sex education controversy that bore signs of common origin was a letter used by foes of sex education throughout the country. In one community after another, often thousands of miles apart, this letter began to appear on school officials' desks. It usually began,

> You are hereby notified that _____ is not allowed by the undersigned to participate in, or be subject to instruction in, any training or education in sex and / or sexual attitudes, human and animal reproductive biological development, introspective examination of social and cultural aspects of family life, or group therapy of self-criticism or any combination or degree thereof, without the consent of the undersigned by express written permission.

Then after including every form of communication, direct or indirect, under the prohibition, the writer usually closed by saying that if the child must be removed from the class to protect him from his sort of thing, then ". . .any damage to the child— emotional or otherwise—caused by this separation shall be deemed the responsibility of the parties to whom this notice is sent."[31]

Precisely what was left for the teacher to do after complying with this directive is not clear. But the scope and character of the list of exclusions suggests that it must have had little to do with critical thinking.

Meanwhile, Gordon Drake and his "Crusade" compatriots continued to stump the country agitating and organizing. Only now they had the help of the John Birch Society, and of many other Rightist groups, all of which were pushing the theme of sex, SIECUS, and subversion.

5

Mopping up

The "antis" get results

As the 1968–69 school year progressed the controversy grew more and more intense. Local committees of "concerned parents" proliferated and opposition to sex education continued to mount. The true believers of the Radical Right became thoroughly commingled with a bewildering array of opponents that ranged from borderline psychotics to responsible professionals. And the unreason, fear, and suspicion that Drake and other zealots had pumped in contributed to an atmosphere of bitter acrimony.

There was a slight lull in the controversy during the summer of 1969 and then the whole controversy took off again as the school bells rang that autumn. By Christmas recess the controversy was even greater than the year before and some of the "antis" pressure was producing some very tangible results.

One of the easiest results to tally was on the legislative front. California and New York passed laws that restricted sex education. Alabama, Delaware, Florida, Illinois, Iowa, Louisiana, Michigan, New Jersey, North Carolina, Pennsylvania, Tennessee, Washington, and Wisconsin were considering resolutions, investigations, or bills that would prohibit, control, or investigate sex education.

Similar bills had been introduced in Arizona, Minnesota, Nevada, and Oklahoma but had become lost in committee.[1]

Two State boards of education had also taken action during 1969. Nebraska's board passed a resolution warning local boards of the dangers of the SIECUS program. The California board passed a resolution expressly prohibiting SIECUS material in the schools.[2]

In a speech in Arlington, Virginia, on the 20th of February, 1969, Drake boasted of forming ". . .a State group" in California. He added, "We worked with the assistance of the Board of Education and that was back in November." He vocally pondered "Should we discuss these things out in the open?" and then said ". . .the State Board of California is investigating the programs in the State of California and we played a very integral part of [sic] this act."[3]

How much of this was puffery and how much fact is difficult to determine. But the fact that Dr. Max Rafferty was California's Superintendent of Schools and Ronald Reagan is Governor makes it at least plausible.

In the Congress of the United States, Representative Henry C. Schadeberg (R., Wisconsin) introduced a bill that would withhold Federal funds from sex education courses or related teacher training. And Representative Rarick introduced a bill calling for a Congressional investigation of SIECUS.[4]

It is much more difficult to take stock of the impact of the anti–sex education campaign at the local level. There is simply no way of telling how many programs were either damaged or aborted in the thousands of local school districts across the country. And even if we could tally known cases, how could we ever determine how many principals or superintendents quietly shelved the possibility of such a program as not worth the "hassle" or took refuge behind the "anti" campaign as an excuse for their own ennui. Further, one cannot help but speculate on the plight of teachers already engaged in teaching children about even their biological, let alone their fully sexual, nature. How many of them quietly backed off?

One ominous, albeit rather shaky, indication of local impact is the fact that Abington Township elementary school officials in Abington, Pennsylvania, felt compelled to abandon plans for a Family Life course.[5] Abington Township is an affluent suburb of Philadelphia with a statewide reputation for educational innovation. If a school district with these credentials abandoned its plans, one cannot help but wonder about the impact on more traditionally conservative systems.

Sensitivity training

As was previously mentioned, one of Drake's original contributions to the sex education controversy was his lumping it with sensitivity training.

Mary Calderone has stated that "SIECUS has taken no position on sensitivity training," and that "I've personally written that we need to know a great deal more about this technique before we allow it to proceed indiscriminately."[6]

The NEA freely acknowledges its association with the National Training Laboratories Institute for Applied Behavioral Research and also acknowledges that it has "been studying and teaching sensitivity training since 1947."[7]

However, the NEA views it as ". . .a learning technique. . . whereby a person can become more sensitive and aware of his real self, and can learn to understand interpersonal relationships and communicate with his fellow man."[8]

Of course, sensitivity training would be a particularly valuable teaching tool in a Family Life and Sex Education Course. But the NTL and the NEA have both been emphatic in stating that sensitivity training must be used judiciously, that it should be avoided by persons with severe emotional troubles, that is is not a group therapy session, and not "an extension of the phychiatrist's couch."[9] Additionally, the NTL has always maintained that sensitivity sessions must be conducted by thoroughly qualified teachers and that it is definitely not something a teacher should attempt with his class. Rather, ideally, the teacher would draw upon the experience for further self-understanding and understanding of the behavior and problems of his pupils.[10]

Despite the ready availability of these facts, Dr. Drake constantly pushed the notion that sensitivity training ". . .is an insidious methodology which aims to destroy the traditional Hebraic-Christian morality of America,"[11] that it was part and parcel of family life and sex education, and that it was all of a piece with naval gazing, nude marathons, Communist "brain washing," and the like.[12]

The NEA has observed that sex and sensitivity do have at least two things in common. "They both begin with the same letter and there are many people who don't know much about either of them."[13] In this context, it is a tribute to Gordon Drake's ingenuity and involvement in the controversy that his curious notions regarding sensitivity training rode about on the back of the sex education battle nearly everywhere that it went.

The "anti" campaign peaks

During the 1968–69 school year the sex education controversy emerged from relative obscurity to rival integration as the pedagogical issue of the decade. The populace was obviously "bullish" for this sort of thing and no one knows how many educators were caught unprepared in the stampede.

During the summer lull the Radical Rightists prepared for an even bigger year in 1969–70. And for a while it looked as if they would be equally successful; only later did it become apparent that some new variables had already begun altering the odds.

For one thing, the NEA had launched a counterattack. Their method consisted chiefly of informing the press, public, and schools as to the Radical Rightist origin of much of the attack.

This informational campaign was formalized in March of 1970, when the controversy was at an all-time high, with the introduction of a booklet, *Suggestions for Defense Against Extremist Attack: Sex Education in the Public Schools.*[14] By September of 1969 this booklet had achieved fairly wide circulation and many teachers, administrators, and school board members had a better idea of the nature of their adversary and the tactics that he employed.

The previous year's controversy had also put school authorities on their guard. In many cases, they had gained time to back off from what they had been doing or indefinitely postpone what they had been planning. In fact, the sudden fall-off in the popularity of the anti–sex education movement probably had more to do with the schools either scrapping or watering down their courses than anything else.

Ironically, by concentrating their attacks on SIECUS the Fund-radists inadvertently provided school authorities with a very effective way of defusing the issue. For if the schools learned nothing else during the 1968–69 battle, they learned that any association with SIECUS meant trouble. Thus, by simply avoiding even the hint of connection with this organization educators deprived the Radical Right of their primary weapon.[15]

The exposés begin

Another important new variable to enter the picture was a better-informed citizenry. Throughout the spring of 1969 there were some rather desultory efforts on the part of minor segments of the mass media to inform the public about the Radical Right's role in the controversy. But, for one reason or another, the major publications which had so eagerly announced the onrush of sex education programs remained silent when the time came to defend the trend from extremist attack.

This changed dramatically at the beginning of the new school year. In September, *Look, Life,* and *Redbook* all published articles on the controversy. And all three of them charged the Radical Right with exploiting the issue through the encouragement of wild distortions and outright lies.[16]

Look recounted how a "savage fight" over sex education had erupted in "more than 34 states across the U.S."[17] The magazine reported that in June 1969 a Gallup poll showed seventy-one percent of adults questioned in favor of sex education in the schools, then asked "Why the fuss?" Their answer was the activities of the Birch Society and the Christian Crusade. *Look* noted how two widely separate communities, Anaheim and Watkins Glen, New York, had been torn apart by the controversy and a bitter residue left behind, despite the fact that such respected groups as the American Medical Association, the National Education Association, the Congress of Parents and Teachers, the National Council of Churches, and many other professional organizations had endorsed school-based sex education as a valuable activity. And the magazine laid the blame on ". . .the scurrilous literature, the wild stories, and the misrepresentations circulated by the Birchers and similar groups. . . ."[18]

Life noted how parents had been ". . .egged on by (the) right-wing Christian Crusade and John Birch Society. . ." and spiked three of the rightists' spiciest rumors.[19]

Redbook did an extensive article which debunked rumor after rumor while pointing the finger of guilt at ". . .a handful of far-right-wing organizations that have a record of attempting to force unrepresentative and often bizarre opinions on the nation's schools."[20] The magazine called specific attention to activities of the John Birch Society, the Christian Crusade, and Dr. Gordon V. Drake and showed how they were allied. It denounced ". . .a return to the tactics of the late Senator Joseph McCarthy,"[21] pointed out innocent men hurt by the unreasoning hate and fear, and summed up by saying,

> Smear sheets and scare tactics by emotionally overwrought individuals and groups do a grave disservice to those teachers, administrators and parents who are sincerely giving of their personal time and energy in an attempt to work together for an improved educational program for our children.[22]

In October 1969, the *Reader's Digest* ran a similar exposé. Like *Redbook* it divulged the cooperative roles of Christian Crusade, Drake, and the Birch Society and demonstrated how "the same material appears in city after city; the same techniques and arguments are used across the country."[23] As for the charges of communist affiliations, the *Digest* said, "If the charges. . .weren't so vicious, they would be almost amusing."[24] And to suggest that the *Reader's Digest* has pinko tendencies would be to overreach even the audacity of Robert Welch.

Look, Life, Redbook, and *Reader's Digest* reached a pretty broad spectrum—including most teachers. So the Radical Right had little cover left. And to make matters worse, *Good Housekeeping* in November came up with the most thorough investigative reporting job of them all.[25]

Drake resigns

Meanwhile, things were not going well at Crusade Headquarters. On the 13th of November, 1969, Dr. Gordon V. Drake announced his resignation as Educational Director of the Christian Crusade and his plans to open a new college in Milwaukee.[26]

Drake's resignation, encouraged by Hargis,[27] reportedly had to do with his unwillingness to "back off" from a Tulsa public school unit which sought to prevent sex education in any form.

Whether this was the real reason for the breakup is hard to say. Since they were being hit by one exposé after another, Hargis may have decided to adopt a low profile and Drake refused. On the other hand, Drake may have seen that the auxiliary cause was drying up and that he should move at the peak of his notoriety. In any event, his parting marked the diminution of the "anti" campaign to an eventual whimper. And only one month after Drake's departure Hargis announced a fifty percent decline in the Crusade's income.[28]

The anticlimax

Of course, the forces that Capell and Drake had set in motion did not simply disappear. Ironically, just two months after Drake's departure, Paul Cook, the superintendent of the Anaheim Union High School District, was forced to resign—shortly after the FLSE program had been suspended, Cook charged ". . .I was forced out by a school board which yielded to a deliberate campaign by a noisy minority."[29]

In a February 1970 "Hargis Letter" Billy James boasted of the Christian Crusade's role in ousting Paul Cook and sought to use his ouster as a springboard for a new sex campaign centering on his own book *The Sex Revolution in the United States.*

But largely as a result of the exposure of the Radical Right's methods during the anti–sex education campaign, Paul Cook was popularly regarded more as the innocent scapegoat of extremists than as a red-tainted archvillain. Hargis' efforts reached no farther than his standard audience.

Court suits against sex education were still pending in a number of states. Oklahoma, Georgia, Idaho, Kentucky, and West Virginia saw their legislators consider bills that would prohibit, control or investigate sex education[30] and countless "true believers" held on to their local school officials like grim death. But the controversy was diminishing and nothing the Radical Right could muster would bring it to full vitality again.

In retrospect

The Chrstian Crusade is still involved in anti–sex education activities, the latest organizational device being the "National Council of Christian Families Opposed to Sex Education in Public Schools." But the effort is desultory at best and the rest of the Radical Right is looking elsewhere.

The bitter and antagonistic controversy has left its own ugly legacy. Legitimate doubts and complaints regarding sex education were never really debated. Many school systems have suspended, curtailed, postponed, or cancelled their sex education or family life programs and are fearful of reviving them. SIECUS is more cautious. Requests for information from schools are at a low ebb and the organization has turned its attention elsewhere. And a SIECUS spokesman said "Had the campaign not existed we probably would have come out with something for the kids."[31]

There are several important general conclusions that also remain to be drawn from the struggle. First, the sex education controversy clearly illustrated the interlocking network of cooperation that exists within the Radical Right and includes the Fundradists. But no "conspiratorial network" theory need be built on this. The evidence suggests that if an auxiliary cause catches on, the rest of the Right jumps aboard. Moreover, this "jumping-aboard" is probably hindered almost as much by petty jealousy as it is aided by common goals.

Insofar as education is concerned, this controversy vividly demonstrated that the Fundradists and the rest of the Radical Right can really "swing a lot of clout" so long as they are complaining about things that touch public nerves. And this effect is heightened by the low voter turnout standard in school elections.[32] By themselves they amount to little so far as a national force is concerned, but when combined with frightened, misinformed citizens they have demonstrated themselves capable of raising educational dust about as high as it has gotten in the last forty or fifty years.[33]

section 2

Leaders, organizations, resources, and methods

6

Carl McIntire's
Twentieth Century
Reformation

I f we use the criteria of length of involvement and degree of exposure to public knowledge, Carl McIntire ranks first in the Fundradist order of things. From its very beginning as a distinguishable entity in American Protestantism, the Fundradist movement has borne his signature. He nurtured it, shaped it, set its ideological tone, established its major leaders, and set the direction if its thrust.[1]

Because of McIntire's position of leadership and central importance in the history of the movement, we will devote a greater amount of attention to his history and current activities than to those of any other. This emphasis serves several purposes. First, it concentrates our attention on that portion of the movement that has the greatest potential for giving us broad understanding. Second, it is the most logical way of introducing those movements, second only to McIntire's in importance, which resulted from the efforts of men that he introduced to the business. Finally, because many of the important details involve the early part of this century, it helps to complete the historical information detailed in Chapter 12, which concludes with the end of the nineteenth century.

The beginning

For more than forty of his sixty-four years "Dr." Carl McIntire has been deeply involved in a peculiar mixture of creation, contention and schism.[2] It began in 1929 when McIntire was a twenty-three-year-old ministerial student at Princeton Theological Seminary. Long a stronghold of the conservative wing of Presbyterianism, the school was being convulsed by the same bitter struggle between Fundamentalists and Modernists that had gripped much of American Protestantism for better than a quarter of a century. But by this time the Fundamentalists were in general retreat and the Princeton conflict took on the air of desperation characteristic of a last stand.

Dr. J. Gresham Machen, a well-known Fundamentalist teacher and author at Princeton, had taken the lead in challenging the presence of modernism at the seminary. Simply stated, it was Machen's contention that the Modernists did not accept the divine authority of the Bible. He took this to be evidence that they rejected the very foundation of Christian faith. He further argued that the Bible was either the word of God or no more than a book of Jewish mythology and that there was no way around this simple fact. Consequently, it followed that a true believer could make no accommodation with Modernism.[3]

Following the dictates of his reasoning, Machen organized sympathetic members of the faculty and student body to banish Modernism from the premises. McIntire was one of his most active student partisans.[4]

Polarization and angry controversy followed Machen's move. In fact, it led to such a disruption of the educative process at the seminary that the Presbyterian Church of the U.S.A. felt compelled to investigate. When the inquiry was completed, the school was reorganized under a more liberal governing board and the right of Modernists to teach or learn at the seminary was firmly established. Machen and his followers were defeated.

Rather than accommodate this reversal, Machen and his sympathizers, including Carl McIntire, left Princeton and established their own seminary in Philadelphia. They called it Westminster. Naturally, it operated on the "no accommodation" principle formulated by Machen. Gritting their teeth, the Presbyterians U.S.A. sanctioned the move.

McIntire graduated from the newly formed school in 1931, a product of traditional Presbyterianism's angry reaction to change. Much like the newly commissioned Captain of a refitted but obsolete ship, McIntire slid proudly, but backward, down the ordinational ways—launching a curious career of bailing frantically against the times.

Defrocking and the subsequent creation of the Presbyterian Church of America

Not long after McIntire's ordination, Machen became involved in another struggle—this one designed to expunge Modernism from Presbyterian foreign mission work. When this failed he organized an Independent Board of Foreign Missions. This paralleled the official board and sought to take over its function. The now "Reverend" McIntire was a charter member.

In 1934 the Presbyterian Church ordered the rival board to cease operation. When they refused, churchly judicial action was started. It culminated in 1936 with the defrocking of Machen, McIntire, and five others for "defaming the character of fellow Christians, breaking certain of the Ten Commandments, causing 'dissension and strife' and 'engendering suspicions and ill will.' "[5] Machen and his followers countered by forming a new denomination—the Presbyterian Church of America.

Collingswood Church

Meanwhile, the large and strongly Fundamentalist Collingswood, New Jersey, Presbyterian Church had appointed the youthful but already controversial Carl McIntire as its pastor. When the defocking came, the church chose to remain loyal to McIntire and withdrew from the Presbyterian Church of the U.S.A.

A dispute arose over ownership of the church. After a bitter struggle the matter went to civil court where McIntire and his church members lost. Undaunted, they rented a circus tent and, under the watchful eye of the news media, they solemnly paraded from the old church into the canvas edifice while singing "Savior Like a Shepherd Lead Us."[6]

Oscar Wilde is reputed to have said that "The only bad publicity you can get is your own obituary." Over the years McIntire has exhibited a penchant for publicity that betrays a likely appreciation of Wilde's view. Certainly, since this event, which paid off handsomely so far as advertising his cause was concerned, McIntire has perfected the technique of turning reversals to advantage by gaining publicity that has the potential of portraying him as one who is enduring persecution for the sake of his beliefs. Actually, in this respect, McIntire has gone Wilde one better. In January 1970 he obtained a copy of an advance obituary written about him by the Associated Press. Since the obituary was not particularly flattering, McIntire seized the opportunity to bemoan its "bias" and declare it to be a prime example of the smear tactics of the "liberal press." He declared that God had "placed the document in his hands" in order to prove how the press was "manipulating" the public. He also conjured up images of his wife reading it while preparing for his burial and of himself rising from the casket to confront his wrongdoers. He broadcast this around the world.[7]

Today, thirty-eight years after his appointment as pastor, McIntire is still in that pulpit; though his circus tent now stands replaced by a modern church and Sunday School complex valued at close to one million dollars[8] and claiming a membership of 1,800.[9]

Architecturally this complex reveals the Fundradists' ideological mixing of religion and nationalism which will be detailed in Chapter 10. It bears a deliberate resemblance to Independence Hall.[10]

Though his operations are large and diverse, Carl McIntire's Collingswood Church is still a nucleus of his activities. It is from here that he has expanded and it has been in this direction that he has retreated when the going has gotten tough. However, his present popularity, coupled with the number of alternative organizational nuclei that he now has available, makes McIntire less dependent on this church than he has been in the past.

"Christian liberty" and the birth of the Bible Presbyterians

Not long after the defrocking, McIntire and his followers affiliated with Machen's Presbyterian Church of America. But this union was no sooner joined that it was ripped apart again—a consequence of internal disagreement.

It will be recalled that Machen advocated total separation from those who did not accept the Bible entirely as the word of God. He did, however, readily accept those who disagreed with him regarding matters of interpretation. He also maintained that those within the faith should have sufficient "Christian liberty" to decide for themselves if they were going to smoke, drink, gamble, participate in modern dancing, go to motion pictures, and the like.[11]

Significantly, McIntire disagreed with his teacher on both these counts. First, his line of separation was far more restrictive. He felt that accepting the Bible as the literal word of God was not enough and pushed for the adoption of eschatologically based distinctions, such as premillennialism as opposed to postmillennialism. (Premillennialists maintain that Christ will actually return to earth after the Last Judgment and reign over the millennium—a thousand years of sinless bliss. Postmillennialists maintain that the preaching of the Gospel will bring about the millennium and that Christ will physically come bringing the Last Judgment at its end.) Second, McIntire was against allowing believers the freedom to choose between drinking and not drinking, smoking and not smoking, and so forth. Instead, he demanded pledges of abstinence from seminary faculty, students, candidates for the mission fields, and practicing clergy. This ran counter to Machen's desire for "Christian liberty" within the denomination and simultaneously antagonized many potential allies—including a goodly number who did none of these things but resented the idea of an oath or pledge.[12]

These differences between McIntire and Machen tore the Presbyterian Church of America in two. Predictably, the most dogmatic faction lined up with McIntire and formed the Bible Presbyterian denomination. Machen died of pneumonia in 1937 while touring the nation, desperately trying to restore the unity that McIntire had destroyed. His followers formed the Orthodox Presbyterians shortly after his death.

McIntire and his small band of Bible Presbyterians were left very much alone in 1938—isolated not only from the mainstream of American Protestantism, but from the vast majority of Fundamentalists as well. What is more, Westminster Seminary, the only facility of the now-fragmented denomination that offered any real organizational leverage, had gone to the Orthodox half of the split.[13] All that remained for the Bible Presbyterians to build from was the Collingswood Church, a newborn, tabloid style religious newspaper, a small band of dogmatic dedicated followers, and the charismatic leadership of Carl McIntire. But that was to prove sufficient to furnish the beginnings of his "Twentieth Century Reformation"—the chief spawning ground for the Fundradist movement.

The Christian Beacon

In 1936, a year before the Presbyterian Church of America split, McIntire founded the *Christian Beacon*—a weekly, eight-page, tabloid style religious newspaper. During the power struggle that preceded the split the paper became McIntire's principal means of partisan persuasion and disputation.[14]

Born in the hostile world of ideologically based schism, the paper alternately assumed the defensive posture of the prey or the aggressive pose of the predator. But whatever the pose, the basic thrust was always highly partisan and reflective of McIntire's thinking.

Building a movement requires an efficient means of mass communication, and the *Christian Beacon* provided McIntire with that tool. With it he spread the word of his exclusivist doctrine, winning new converts, and while gaining the resources required to win still more, it set an important precedent. For when McIntire moved from pulpit to print shop and found what he needed, it convinced him that a Twentieth Century Reformation would require its leader to utilize modern means of mass communication. And this conviction eventually led him to the radio studio and the real beginning of his mass popularity.

Although supplanted in importance by McIntire's radio broadcasts, the *Christian Beacon* is still very much alive. McIntire is Editor-in-Chief; and with a claimed circulation of 123,000, it remains his principal means of communication via the printed word.[15]

Characteristically, the paper makes heavy use of the "documented appraisal" technique. This involves reprinting articles from various sources, frequently without permission, and then subjecting them to comment or rebuke. But even the casual reader would not interpret this style as an attempt at objectivity. For the unmistakable thrust of the tabloid is the dissemination of ideologically derived conclusions and these conclusions are clearly those of Carl McIntire.

A surprising amount of material critical of Carl McIntire or his movement is reprinted in the *Christian Beacon*. However, close examination reveals that particularly telling blows are either ignored or reproduced in an incomplete fashion (e.g., only the first and often least damaging page).[16]

The *Christian Beacon* also served as the organizational base for the formation of the Twentieth Century Reformation's own publishing company. Known as the Christian Beacon Press, this company provides a means of publication for material produced by organizations that are part of McIntire's movement. It has also been the means of publishing all of Carl McIntire's many books and tracts.[17]

Achievement of control

McIntire was hurt by his split with Machen. The most serious damage resulted from the loss of Westminster Seminary and the profound alienation of many previous allies who now tended to regard him as an ungrateful opportunist who had stabbed his mentor in the back. In fact, of the 128 ministers who had affiliated themselves with the Presbyterian Church of America, only 31 withdrew to go McIntire's way.[18]

But despite the cost, McIntire had achieved the creation of a denominationally based movement whose ideological and organizational thrust was not blunted by internal divisiveness. What is more, there was no longer any question of sharing power. So far as the "ultra" faction of Presbyterianism's revolt against modernity was concerned, that power was now in the hands of Carl McIntire.

Faith Theological Seminary

The first order of business was the creation of a seminary to replace Westminster. And this was done with surprising speed. Utilizing the *Christian Beacon,* the Collingswood Church, and the churches that had come away with him when the Presbyterian Church of America split, McIntire had a seminary operating in Wilmington, Delaware, before the year was out. They called it Faith Theological Seminary. And although it began with only twenty-four students, new ministers could now be trained for Bible Presbyterian pulpits and the ideology had a safe place to grow.[19]

In 1952 the seminary moved from Wilmington to its present location in a mansion in Elkins Park, Pennsylvania, a suburb of Philadelphia. This property includes some choice suburban acreage that could be worth as much as ten million dollars.[20]

As president of its board, McIntire exercised considerable influence over the seminary, though until recently his control was incomplete. For example, McIntire's 1969 ouster from the Board of Directors of Christian Churches revealed he had some bitter enemies within the seminary. McIntire's alienated colleague, Dr. John Millheim, general secretary of the ACCC, quotes one anonymous member of the faculty as saying to him, "You either have to look at what he [McIntire] is doing as [the actions of] a man who has visions of grandeur to the point where he feels that he is an incarnate prophet, or [decide] that is is an evil man. After evaluating that situation for more than twenty years, I would say that he is a very evil man."[21]

This dissension within the seminary broke into the open in 1971. At this time Dr. Allan MacRae, president of the seminary for thirty-seven years, all but two faculty members, and more than half of the students quit. This walkout was a direct result of a struggle between Dr. MacRae and the pro-McIntire Board of Directors. The struggle had its immediate origins in Dr. McIntire's "dictatorial" style, his efforts to organize political rallies demanding "total victory" in Indochina, and the "crude and disagreeable methods" of ". . .a small group of students" who ". . . made themselves utterly obnoxious. . ." by carrying on a ". . . campaign for every single word Dr. McIntire might utter on any subject. . . ."[22]

The walkout left McIntire with little more than the building. But he quickly regrouped, hired new faculty of more personal loyalties, and had himself installed as president. Then he pronounced that the seminary had been ". . .indeed delivered to be a greater part of the Twentieth Century Reformation Movement over the whole world."[23]

The "deliverance" may be of short duration. The seminary went into debt to buy radio station WXUR in order that Dr. McIntire might air his views. In a landmark decision upheld by the courts, this station was denied license renewal on the ground that it violated the Fairness Doctrine and attempted to deceive a Federal regulatory body. This placed the seminary in financial jeopardy. (Details concerning this denial of license renewal appear later in this chapter.)

The Bible Presbyterians oust McIntire

After establishing Faith Theological Seminary, McIntire set the organizational sights of the Bible Presbyterians higher. Soon they had gone on to establish a home for the aged, a summer Bible conference and two small colleges—Shelton in Cape May, New

Jersey, and Highland in Pasadena, California. (The latter has since closed after a struggle for its control.) Meanwhile, the number of congregations affiliating with the denomination rose steadily. Eventually the Bible Presbyterians claimed over one hundred member churches. But in 1956 a dispute that had been smoldering for some time burst into flame. A large group of dissatisfied member churches angrily charged that McIntire was "undemocratic" in his style of leadership. Further, they claimed that he was too involved in other activities to give the job the attention it deserved. Finally, they charged that he was guilty of grossly inflating Bible Presbyterian membership figures.[24] These grievances, coupled with McIntire's subsequent refusal to accommodate the dissidents, led to open revolt.

The anti-McIntire faction constituted a majority of the members of the denomination and they had little difficulty gaining control of its organizational apparatus. When this was accomplished McIntire was unceremoniously dumped. For good measure the denomination also voted themselves out of the American and International Councils of Christian Churches—two organizations founded by McIntire. No more than twenty percent of the churches remained loyal to McIntire.[25] The rest joined in his ouster. There could be little question that he and his cause were badly hurt.

But McIntire still controlled the Collingswood Church—the largest in the denomination. What was more, those loyal to him continued to control Faith Seminary and the *Christian Beacon*. Using this base McIntire reorganized his remaining followers and declared that they were the real representatives of Bible Presbyterianism.[26]

For several confusing years there were two Bible Presbyterian denominations—the original and McIntire's second creation. McIntire's endurance eventually proved the greater. In 1961 the original organization finally changed its name to the Evangelical Presbyterian Church.[27]

But winning the battle of the names did not mean that McIntire had won the war. As a matter of fact, the denomination has been anemic ever since the revolt. Current membership hovers around the 8,000-mark, making the Bible Presbyterians a minuscule part of American Protestantism.[28]

Founding of the American Council of Christian Churches

Had McIntire been content to rest on his laurels after founding the Bible Presbyterian denomination this revolt could well have smashed his "Twentieth Century Reformation" movement. But, far from relaxing after his first major success, McIntire had been very busy developing other bases of support. Consequently, he and his cause survived with surprisingly little damage.

One of the most important of these "other bases of support" was the American Council of Christian Churches, established under McIntire's leadership in 1941. Representing the broadest national base of ecclesiastical support that McIntire's "Reformation" has ever secured, this council eventually attracted fifteen denominations with a combined membership of 200,000 to 250,000.[29]

One of the primary motivations for founding the ACCC was to counter the growing power of the newly created Federal (now National) Council of Churches. The formation of the Federal Council represented the first time that American Protestantism had been able to effect any meaningful measure of interdenominational cooperation. Such an accomplishment, however roughhewn at the start, represented a very real change in the various member denominations' devotion to their own dogma and, more importantly, the feeble beginnings of ecumenism.

Naturally, such a course of events was viewed with profound alarm by those elements of American Protestantism whose belief structures were rigidly doctrinaire. And nowhere was the alarm greater than among those denominations representing the "ultra" fringe of Fundamentalism; for they were the most rigid and doctrinaire of them all.

Carl McIntire took the alarm of these "ultras" and gave it organizational structure by creating the American Council of

Christian Churches. He was considerably aided in this endeavor by the national notoriety that he had gained while championing the cause of "total separation" and by his ability to use the *Chrisian Beacon* as an instrument of persuasion.

Soon he had gathered a small band of zealots who believed that they alone represented the posture of defenders of the faith and denouncers of apostasy, and they waxed continously indignant over the fact that the ACCC was not treated with the same interest and deference as the giant Federal Council. This attitude persisted despite the fact that the Federal Council outnumberd them by about 168 to 1; and despite the even more devastating fact that American Fundamentalism was more accurately represented by the National Association of Evangelists, which McIntire had refused to join and which enjoyed membership odds of 8 to 1.[30] But mere members mean little or nothing to those who see themselves as the only representatives of good in a world divided between good and evil.

To be sure, those that joined the ACCC were similar to the general run of Fundamentalists in that they insisted on the verbal inspiration of the Bible, Jesus' virgin birth and the other major doctrines of traditional Protestant Orthodoxy. But they were also committed to McIntire's powerful brand of "total separation" and to his stand against "Christian liberty." These commitments, plus the degree of their zeal in the other areas, put them on the "ultra" fringe.

"True believers" tend to dichotomize and to categorize people as belonging to in-groups and out-groups. And this tendency has been quite strong in American Fundamentalism. But McIntire's doctrine of "total separation" was so severe in its dichotomization that even the majority of Fundamentalists were put off by it.

Similarly, Fundamentalism is built on the notion that faith and salvation can be defined in terms of a one-hundred-percent commitment to certain "absolute truths." Such a belief suggests that it is both possible and permissible to coerce men into accepting such a commitment as was done in the Inquisition. However, such coercion has never set well with most American Protestants, probably due to the nation's philosophical commitment to individual freedom and the necessities imposed by pluralism.[31] Ironically, considering his devotion to "patriotic" causes, McIntire apparently suffered no such discomfort when contemplating coercion. By demanding that Machen's commitment to "Christian liberty" be abandoned he adopted a position that ignored the tension between commitment to exclusive "absolute truths" and devotion to individual freedom and mutual tolerance. Instead, he defined the problem away by claiming that freedom could only reside within these truths.[32] Here again, even though Fundamentalism's commitment to dogmatic truths predisposed it to be antilibertarian and undemocratic, McIntire simply went too far for most Fundamentalists.

Thus we see that from its very inception the ACCC was not just an anti-Modernist movement. It also embodied a largely unacknowledged, but supremely important, split between McIntire's partisans and the rest of Fundamentalism that has its origin in the essentially undemocratic and antilibertarian nature of McIntire's emerging ideology. He was clearly moving in the direction of demanding that individuals conform to his particular interpretation of a supreme imperative even though this required a disregard for American political ideals.[33] The average Fundamentalist was simply not ready to buy this.

Official parting

This divergence became official in 1942 when informal negotiations were begun in St. Louis, Missouri, to explore the possibility of organizing all of the nation's conservative Protestants in opposition to the Federal Council. As the President of the ACCC, McIntire made it clear that he would cooperate in this endeavor only if the principle of "total separation" were adhered to. No member would be permitted to have anything to do with the Federal Council.[34]

Although the delegates shared McIntire's antipathy to the Federal Council, they believed that individuals should have the freedom to choose between resisting apostasy within the Federal

Council and totally withdrawing from it.[35] But, true to form, McIntire would not compromise the "total separation" principle in deference to individual liberty. Consequently, he withdrew from the discussions. The majority that remained went on to establish the National Association of Evangelicals, the organization that has come to represent the mainstream of America's Fundamentalist Protestantism.

Founding of the International Council of Christian Churches

In 1948, McIntire established still another base of support when he organized the International Council of Christian Churches. Like the American Council, this organization was based on angry backlash to the growing ecumenism of Protestant Christianity— in this case on an international scale.

When the World Council of Churches scheduled its first meeting for Amsterdam in 1948, McIntire arranged a simultaneous convocation in the same city and set up the International Council. McIntire's meeting was a miniscule affair that Donald Barnhouse, editor and founder of the Fundamentalist-oriented *Eternity* magazine, described at the time as "a side show that finished in fiasco."[36] But the tactic employed produced reams of publicity and McIntire has since adopted a standard policy of organizing rival meetings every time an important Protestant ecumenical-style meeting is convened.[37]

McIntire was president of the ACCC for only one year. But he has been the president of the International Council since its founding. Additionally, its headquarters were established in McIntire's own Twentieth Century Reformation building.[38] Perhaps McIntire set up his own control in this firm fashion because he was already experiencing difficulties in controlling the ACCC. But whatever the motivation, it was to prove to be a wise policy for he would eventually be forced to retreat to this position.

McIntire claims that the ICCC has grown to represent eighty-nine sects with over one million members.[39] But members of his own organization alleged that he inflated ACCC membership figures, so this figure may be inaccurate. It will suffice to say that compared to the mammoth World Council of Churches, the International Council is and always has been minuscule.

Extension of McIntire's ideology and the advent of the Cold War

By the end of the Second World War it looked as if the Federal Council and the National Association of Evangelists were going to be able to accommodate the pressures of the times without provoking their followers to join McIntire's movement. His "Twentieth Century Reformation" was making little headway.

But a shift in McIntire's ideology and a related change in international politics were destined to reverse the trend. The shift in ideology involved the extension of McIntire's theology into the political and economic realms.[40] The change in international politics involved the advent of the Cold War.

The birth of modern Fundamentalism coincided with the advent of the First World War, when religious nationalism was near the peak of its popularity. It had consolidated its position during the "Great Red Scare" of the early 1920s. Both of these times left their marks on the movement and Fundamentalism came to include a measure of "Christian-Americanism" and ill-defined "Anti-Communism" as an integral part of its ideology.[41]

These influences came to their first fruition during the 1930s, when men such as the Rev. Gerald B. Winrod, the Rev. Gerald L. K. Smith, and William Dudley "Chief" Pelley blended Fundamentalism with ultra right-wing or quasi-fascist political activities.[42] But these men had built their movements on the frustrations, anxieties, and alienation of the depression era—using the New Deal as their chief symbol of all that was evil. Consequently, when Roosevelt and the New Deal were overwhelmingly endorsed in the election of 1936, there was little for these predecessors of the Fundradists to do but retire to the hinterlands, lick their wounds, and grow increasingly hysterical as the changing times pressed in on them. Eventually, some of them began to play on anti-Semitic feeling instead of opposition to the New Deal. But this was a fatal mistake. Soon the entire movement came to be identified in the public mind with Nazism and its attendant anti-Semitism, and with the beginning of World War II this movement's power and popularity declined severely.[43] It remained for Carl McIntire to seize the unparalleled opportunity presented by the Cold War in order to really unite the "fundamentalism of the cross" with the "fundamentalism of the flag."[44]

Although he had been moving in this direction for some time, it was not until 1946, with the publication of *Author of Liberty,* that McIntire finally took the step that indicated he had become a full-fledged resident of the Radical Right.[45] Leaning heavily on the shock, disillusion, and confusion that arose when the winning of World War II brought the Cold War instead of peace, McIntire maintained that the Nation's socioeconomic and political systems, in their original, unadulterated forms, were instruments of God's purpose and that it was primarily because the nation had lost sight of this fact that things were going badly. He then proposed that "Communism" was relentlessly exploiting this loss of purpose for Satan—primarily through the cooperation of stupidity of native Americans.[46] And in this fashion the ideology with which we will become more familiar took its shape.

McIntire's *ultra*-Fundamentalism had derived from his desire to totally subordinate the individual to certain "absolute truths" even though this was at odds with the Nation's political ideals. Now we find him joining the ranks of the political extremists by attacking the very logic of American democracy. He did this by proclaiming that democracy's right to exist was solely derived from its usefulness as a means of serving Jesus Christ. Man and society were to be brought to conform to McIntire's vision of the higher goal, a goal that was above the law. America was simply God's tool.[47]

Impact of McCarthyism

At first, this extension of the ideology made little difference in the popularity of McIntire or his organizations. But as the Cold War grew more and more ominous the national climate of opinion began to change. McIntire pounded away with ever-increasing vigor on conspiracy, the "Communist" menace, and the necessity of re-embracing God, the family, and the mythic America of the theocratic "Golden Age." And when this type of approach began to be skillfully used in Congress and the mass media by Senator Joseph R. McCarthy, it became increasingly respectable and popular. Suddenly, McIntire and his followers were on their way to unprecedented public esteem and influence—riding atop a wave of Cold War-engendered, anti-Communistic, one-hundred-percent Americanism.[48]

McIntire had always charged that Modernism and the apostate clergy who had served or coexisted with it were an enormous threat to Christianity and that its "Social Gospel" element slashed at the heart of the American way of life. Now, although he had hinted at "commie" influence before, with the extension of his ideology he really began to push the charge that the nation's churches were riddled with un-American, pro-Communist traitors and their witless dupes.[49]

This fit the thrust of McCarthyism so perfectly that it wasn't long before McIntire and his followers were cooperating directly with Senator McCarthy's staff and that of the House Un-American Activities Committee, by identifying "suspects" within the clergy, a delicate task best left to insiders, and by providing "documentation" on their activities.[50] Being men of the cloth, their presence also provided the proceedings with a very useful touch of divinity. In return, McIntire and his subordinates in the ACCC-ICCC achieved more respectability than they had ever had, while simultaneously gaining a nation-wide forum for their charges. Now the media listened when they charged that the Revised Standard Version of the Bible was the product of a "Red" plot or that the World Council of Churches was a front for "the conspiracy." And most of them reported these allegations in front-page fashion without comment, even when they were obviously and outrageously unfair.[51]

The future Fundradist leaders begin to gather

We have seen how McIntire and his movement were likely rescued from oblivion by the combination of a politicized ideology, the

Cold War and, most of all, McCarthyism. During this same time the religio-political extremists who would later provide the Fundradist movement with its major organizations and leadership began to gather around his changing movement.

The first to arrive was Major (Rev.) Edgar C. Bundy. Born in Connecticut in 1915, but reared in Florida, Bundy was graduated from Wheaton College in 1938. In 1941 he joined the Army and was commissioned the following year. In that same year he was ordained a Southern Baptist minister. In 1948 the then Captain Bundy resigned from active duty to become City Editor of the Wheaton, Illinois, *Daily Journal*.[52] (His promotion to Major came in the reserves.)

Bundy soon associated himself with the ACCC and in 1949 he published an article in the *Christian Beacon* which contained the standard components of the emerging Fundradist ideology. Shortly thereafter he joined McIntire's staff as a part-time public relations man and researcher.[53]

A month after joining McIntire, Bundy was invited by Senator Kenneth McKellar to appear before the Senate Appropriations Committee. He testified that if China were allowed to go Communist then Japan, the Philippines, India, Burma, Malaya, and the Dutch East Indies would fall and predicted that North Korea would invade South Korea. When that last piece of birdshot hit the mark, Bundy found himself much in demand as an "expert" lecturer on Communism.[54]

Bundy soon expanded his activities from public relations and research to become McIntire's resident intelligence expert, his (limited) military experience in this area adding luster to the role. As one might expect, he found conspiracy and subversion in a whole host of places, including the Girl Scouts of America.[55] He also headed the ACCC-ICCC delegation to the hearings of the House Un-American Activities Committee on Methodist Bishop Oxnam.[56]

When the McCarthy era ended, Bundy continued to serve on McIntire's staff. But in 1956 the board of directors of the Church League of America, a curious quasi-religious, private, right-wing, intelligence service, appointed Bundy its new executive director.

In this capacity he was to become a major Fundradist leader in his own right.⁵⁷

The twenty-five-year-old Billy James Hargis, an obscure Fundamentalist preacher of the Christian Church, was the next on the scene. Hargis was born in Texarkana, Texas, in 1925, and after graduating from high school he enrolled in Ozark Bible College in Bentonville, Arkansas.⁵⁸ He was ordained before completing his first year of study and left Ozark permanently after only eighteen months. A series of pastorates in small towns in Missouri and Oklahoma followed.⁵⁹

According to his own account, Hargis had been harboring a growing concern over "the twin threats—Communism within the nation and religious apostasy within the churches."⁶⁰ This led him to resign his pastorate in 1950 in order to begin a full-time campaign against these threats.

Shortly thereafter he appeared in Washington, D.C., where he somehow got access to Senator McCarthy. Apparently McCarthy was impressed, for he later commented that his investigations had been helped by "a great preacher, Dr. Billy James Hargis of Tulsa, Oklahoma, who is pastor of a church there and doing outstanding work."⁶¹ [Hargis received an honorary Doctor of Divinity Degree from Defender Seminary in Puerto Rico in 1954. The seminary was founded by the late Rev. Gerald Winrod, who was so pro-German in World War II that he became known as the "Jayhawk Nazi." Precisely why McCarthy would call him "Dr." three years earlier is not clear.]⁶² Within the year Hargis also incorporated Christian Echoes National Ministry as a "religious, nonprofit body." It was this organization that was to be his vehicle in the crusade "for Christ and against Communism."⁶³

Things went slowly for Hargis until 1953. In that year Carl McIntire hired him as a member of his staff. Shortly thereafter Hargis supervised an ACCC-ICCC project: to fly portions of the King James Version of the Bible into Iron Curtain countries on helium-filled balloons.⁶⁴ While the impact of this Bible barrage on its recipients never became clear, Hargis did hit the front pages for the first time. He later described this as "My biggest break so far as promotion is concerned. . . ."⁶⁵

Hargis flew the ACCC-ICCC Bible balloons for another five years, and, because he had broadcast successfully on radio in his last pastorate, he was also placed on the Radio and Audio Film Commission of the International Council. At the same time he was working for his own Christian Echoes National Ministry, broadcasting on his own four-station network.[66] Hargis' use of this media is quite significant for radio broadcasting has since become the Fundradists' primary means of communication, organization, and fund-raising.[67]

In the late 1950s as his own "Christian Crusade" blossomed, Hargis slowly grew away from McIntire. Eventually, he would head a movement which rivaled that of his old employer in terms of income and holdings.

In 1950 Carl McIntire and Dr. T. T. Shields, a Baptist pastor from Toronto, visited Australia. During their stay they became acquainted with Dr. Frederick Charles Schwarz, a man who had gained a reputation as an unusually erudite anti-Communist speaker in his homeland.

Schwarz was born in Brisbane, Australia, in 1913, the son of a successful Jewish businessman who had converted to Christianity. He attended college and obtained degrees in both science and the liberal arts. Then, while lecturing at Queensland Teachers College, he studied medicine; Schwarz graduated from the University of Queensland Medical School in 1944. He set up a practice in medicine and psychiatry in Sydney while serving as a lay preacher in a local Baptist church.[68]

By his own account, Schwarz's anti-Communist activities date from 1940 when he was badly beaten in a debate with a well-known Australian Communist. Shamed by his defeat, Schwarz launched a vigorous self-education program and soon obtained a sufficient level of proficiency to be in demand as a speaker.[69]

McIntire heard him speak while in Australia and was so impressed by his combination of scholarly acumen and old style evangelistic fervor that he invited him on a two-month lecture tour of America under the sponsorship of the ACCC. The tour enjoyed considerable success.[70]

Schwarz returned to the U.S. in 1952.[71] This time he stayed, setting up his tax-exempt Christian Anti-Communism Crusade in Waterloo, Iowa, with the help of a local radio evangelist and "a group of local Christian men."[72] His stated objectives were

> To combat Communism by means of lectures in schools, colleges, civic clubs, servicemen's organizations and other similar organizations and through radio and television broacasts and by providing courses for missionaries and others to be used in Bible schools and seminaries and the holding of religious and evangelistic services in churches, and through publication of books, pamphlets and literature and by all other appropriate means.[73]

Schwarz's most successful activity was to prove to be his series of traveling "schools" on anti-Communism which have been held all over the nation.[74]

What was to become the central core of Fundradist leadership and activities had now begun to coalesce—all with considerable assistance from Carl McIntire and his Twentieth Century Reformation movement. Edgar Bundy of the Church League of America, Billy James Hargis of the Christian Crusade and Dr. Frederick Schwarz of the Christian Anti-Communist Crusade; all of them grew and prospered in the right-wing hatchery of McCarthyism while finding comfort and assistance under Carl McIntire's organizational wing.

Price of the ideological extension and McIntire's style of leadership

Even though McIntire's cause generally profited from the extension of his ideology into the political and economic realms, the transition was not without cost. Elements within both the ACCC and ICCC were discomfited by the change and by the new activities that it engendered. Additionally, McIntire's egotistical style of leadership rankled many.[75] In 1952 the Evangelical Methodist Church quit the ACCC and the Orthodox Presbyterians withdrew from the ICCC. In 1953 the Independent Fundamental Churches of America severed their relations with the American Council.[76]

The extension of the ideology and McIntire's manner of leadership also had something to do with McIntire's previously described ouster as head of the Bible Presbyterians and their subsequent withdrawal from both councils. Additionally, though the ideological change was gradual and blended nicely with national and international events, it must have alienated many individual followers.

But the highest, though most subtle price, incurred in making the ideological change was that McIntire finished the process of cutting himself off from the main body of American thought and practice. Now he and the movements he headed were not only on the "ultra" fringe of American Protestantism; they were also on the extremist fringe of the nation. In effect, they had finished the process of becoming strangers in their own land.

Hargis points the way

McCarthyism had given an invaluable boost to the emerging Fundradist movtment. But it would be a mistake to think that by the time of McCarthy's fall from grace they had become well-established. What they had become was noticed and to some degree, legitimized. But the maximization of these advantages lay ahead.

At this juncture it was Hargis rather than McIntire who showed the way. In order to make maximum use of the publicity gained in the Bible balloon project, Hargis employed L. E. (Pete) White, the same Tulsa promoter who had helped launch Oral Roberts on his phenomenally successful faith healing campaigns. White's interest was the standard fifteen percent of the gross.[77] Hargis also began making extensive use of his expanding radio ministry and pushing his political and socal views even harder.

Of all the major Fundradist leaders, Hargis, possibly because of his Southern background, made the most direct appeal to anti-Negro prejudice.[78] In the 1950s this emphasis coincided perfectly with the backlash that followed the monumental Supreme Court decision in *Brown* v. *Board of Education* (1954) and the subsequent social upheaval regarding integration and civil rights which blossomed during the latter half of the 1950s.

The combination of White's skillful promotion, the increased use of radio, and Hargis' concentration on racial turmoil as a product of a Communist plot produced major results. In 1955 the Christian Crusade's annual income was approximately $48,400. The Crusade's income in 1956 jumped to approximately $124,000, and by 1957 it was nearing the $171,000 mark.[79]

The "Twentieth Century Reformation Hour" goes on the air

Although his sermons had been broadcast over WCAM in Camden, New Jersey, since 1940, McIntire did not launch his thirty-minute "Twentieth Century Reformation Hour" until 1955. For the first three years of its existence the program was carried on only one station and most of it was devoted to McIntire's blasts against Modernism, the Social Gospel, ecumenism, and other forms of "religious apostasy."[80]

But a change, already reflected in his extended ideology and anticipated by the activities of Billy James Hargis, slowly overtook the program. Increasingly, McIntire began to speak out on national issues rather than the intra-Christian differences, which had once been his primary cause. And as he did, the income and distribution of his program increased dramatically.[81]

In 1958 McIntire began a major expansion of his "new improved" version of the "Twentieth Century Reformation Hour." The Annual Income of the program catapulted from an estimated $62,000 in 1958 to an estimated $1,718,000 in 1963—a nearly 2,700-percent increase in just five years.[82] Additionally, what had started as a one-station daily broadcast in 1955 had expanded to a daily network of a claimed 600 stations,[83] with a mostly rural and suburban audience estimated at near the 20-million mark.[84]

By adopting the twin techniques of emphasizing popular issues and making massive use of radio, Carl McIntire had, after nearly thirty years of trying, finally obtained a medium and a message that enabled him to consistently touch the quick of millions of Americans.[85]

But this success required a very basic alteration in the nature

of the movement itself and, ultimately, the consignment of Mc-
Intire's original "total separation" principle to oblivion.

Emergence of the contemporary
American Radical Right

The sudden success of the "Twentieth Century Reformation Hour"
was remarkable. But this was only part of a more general phenomenon: a major surge in Radical Rightist activity that pulsed
through the entire nation in the late fifties and throughout the
sixties.[86]

McCarthyism never really had a full-fledged ideology, organization, or program that went beyond "anti-Communist" witch hunting.[87] But this new surge soon had all three. Its ideology was the
conspiracy-based, reactionary, "anti-Communist," anti-Democratic
one described in detail in Chapter 11—the overt Fundamentalist
touch being optional. Its organizations were loosely grouped
around Carl McIntire and his activities if the Fundamentalist
Protestant element was overtly present; around the rapidly growing John Birch Society if it was not. Of course, the program was to
work for the implementation of their Radical Rightist ideology.[88]

The blending

In extending his ideology in the postwar 1940s McIntire anticipated the formation of the secular American Radical Right by
more than a decade. Yet even when it became obvious that, according to Erling Jorstad, he and the secular groups were "moving in
the same direction along parallel tracks,"[89] McIntire did not jump
into a union with them.

This wariness had at least some of its origin in the "total
separation" principle. Cooperation with the John Birch-dominated
secular wing of the Radical Right would require either giving up or
drastically modifying this concept. McIntire's past activities indicate a reluctance on his part to join anything that he cannot
ultimately control. His reluctance to join with the secular Radical
Right, and even his "total separation" principle itself, could be

interpreted as having their ultimate origin here. If so, "total separation" becames a function of total egotism.

But Hargis, who had never been associated with the total separation principle historically, was eager to establish liaison with the secular Radical Right and was doing very well indeed. Moreover, a spontaneous trend towards cooperation was creeping in, despite the "total separation" principle, as the state of the nation grew, in Radical Rightist eyes, increasingly desperate.[90]

Finally, when the possibility of electing Senator Barry Goldwater to the Presidency of the United States presented itself in 1964, even the doctrine of "total separation" could not prevent McIntire from joining forces with the secular wing. The opportunity was simply too great to be missed. And so it was that an interlocking, convoluted complex of cooperation between the secular and the religious Radical Right finally formed. The passion of the union suggested that they had been meant for one another all along.[91]

Cape May complex

The success of McIntire's "Twentieth Century Reformation Hour" broadcast brought his movement its first substantial income. Some of this money was put to use in 1962 when the nonprofit Christian Beacon Press, Inc., bought the unused 333-room Admiral Hotel plus adjoining acreage in Cape May, New Jersey, for an estimated $300,000.[92] The hotel was dilapidated, but an extensive renovation, estimated at $250,000, restored it.[93] Today it functions as the heart of a growing "Bible Conference and Freedom Center," where speakers such as the Rev. Ian Paisley, Major Edgar Bundy, and Senator Strom Thurmond may be heard during the summer months.

In 1967 McIntire used the radio to solicit $150,000 as a down payment on the famous 100-room Congress Hall Hotel, an adjacent restaurant, and five surrounding acres at the Cape. Six presidents of the United States had used the Congress Hall during its prime and it was in good repair. The price was $550,000.[94]

In January 1971 McIntire announced the purchase of Cape

May's historic Windsor Hotel, which had been featured in *Life* as one of the "Grand Old Resort Hotels."[95] The purchase price was $230,000.[96]

Cape May was also the site of the "Reformation's" Shelton College until the institution's degree granting rights were revoked by New Jersey as a result of twelve different violations of State standards. It has since moved to McIntire's recently acquired "Freedom Center" in Cape Canaveral, Florida, and the college's new one-million-dollar building in Cape May now stands temporarily idle.[97] But even considering this particular difficulty, Carl McIntire has gone a long way toward turning Cape May into a Radical Rightist's version of Chautauqua.

ACCC's ouster of McIntire and other difficulties

Shelton College's loss of accreditation has not been the only difficulty to beset McIntire's "Reformation." The Federal Communications Commission recently found radio station WXUR in Media, Pennsylvania—owned by Faith Theological Seminary—in violation of the Fairness Doctrine and rejected its application for license renewal. McIntire appealed through the courts; his appeal was resoundingly denied. The United States Court of Appeals found that "During the entire license period Brandywine (WXUR) willfully chose to disregard commission mandate. With more brazen bravado than brains, Brandywine went on an independent frolic broadcasting what it chose, in any terms it chose, abusing those who dared differ with its viewpoints. The record is replete with example after example of one-sided presentation on issues of controversial importance to the public."[98] Significantly, the court also noted that WXUR had practiced "deception" from the moment of its initial license application. In fact, with regard to ". . .candor and honesty in representations to the Commission," the Court observed,

> Their dismal failure in this regard is evidenced in this 8,000-page record. These men, with their hearts bent toward deliberate and premeditated deception, cannot be said to have dealt fairly with the Commission or the people in the Philadelphia area. Their statements constitute a series of heinous misrepre-

sentations which, even without the other factors in this case, would be ample justification for the Commission to refuse to renew the broadcast license.[99]

When the Supreme Court refused to hear McIntire's appeal, he announced his intention to launch a "pirate" radio station that would operate in international waters. At this writing, the ship *Columbia* is standing three and one-half miles off Cape May, New Jersey, preparing to broadcast McIntire's "Radio Free America" message to the Eastern seaboard. The FCC has announced that it will seek a court injunction to halt the broadcasts; the injunction will be based on a broad provision of the Communication Act of 1934.[100]

McIntire has said that he will go to jail, if necessary, in the battle to get his station on the air.[101] Thus the man who has roundly condemned civil disobedience in the most vituperative terms stands ready to use it when his own ox is gored.

Since Faith Seminary mortgaged its property for the purpose of purchasing WXUR, the financial blow to the seminary may be fatal. Further, there is every indication that his radio network is debt-ridden and shrinking. McIntire alleges that this shrinkage is due to fear of FCC censure on the part of the station owners. There is considerable evidence that this is at least partially true.[102]

But his biggest setback to date came when he was repudiated and ousted by his own American Council of Christian Churches. The history of this ouster is entirely too long and involved to cover here. Suffice it to say that the fight broke into the open in 1967 when ACCC leaders alleged that McIntire was using ACCC funds for ICCC purposes.[103]

In 1968 he walked out of the ACCC's Annual Convention in a disagreement over who could attend an executive committee session. In 1969 the ACCC voted to drop McIntire from its executive council. And in 1970, after McIntire attempted to take over that convention during a scheduled recess, creating a huge uproar, the ACCC dropped out of the ICCC and denounced McIntire's actions as "despicable piracy."[104]

It seems likely that much of the ACCC's discontent with McIntire stemmed from anger over his undemocratic style of leadership and his ever-increasing association with political rallies such as the twin "Marches for Victory" held in Washington, D.C., on October 3 and May 8, 1971. John Millheim, general secretary of the ACCC, gave voice to these feelings when he maintained that the "conglomerate crowds" at the rallies violated "the clear and positive commands of God that His people be separate from all unbelief and corruption."[105]

McIntire's "total separation" principle had come full circle. Now *he* was being accused of violating it by associating with non-believers. Thus, as he moved to the political right, McIntire started the process of inadvertently chopping off his religious principles with his political axe.

Cape Canaveral complex

McIntire's ouster from the ACCC did not produce the disastrous results one might have expected. He now had his own church, the radio network, the ICCC, and the Cape May complex to fall back on. But hardly one to rest easy, McIntire launched his most ambitious project to date before the ouster ACCC dust had even cleared: the Cape Canaveral "Freedom Center and Christian Conference."[106] This center included the 200-room, 5-year-old Hilton Hotel, a 2,000-seat convention center, the 260-unit Palm East apartments, the IBM Building, the Brown Engineering Building, the Chrysler Building, and 218 acres of undeveloped real estate. The *assessed* value of the entire complex totals $3,706,070.[107]

The actual price of the total package has not been released, but estimates range from $4 to $25 million.[108] All that Carl McIntire will say is that these properties were "turned over to him" by Shyford Mills and Cevesco, Inc., two corporations represented by businessman H. H. Simms, Jr., "who will remain with Dr. McIntire in an advisory capacity."[109]

Shelton College has relocated in one of the buildings, and plans call for using the remainder of the complex as a "year-round Christian Conference and Freedom Center," as well as a "retirement complex."[110] In short, it is to become a second, and much grander, Cape May.

A last word

We now know something of the way that the Fundradist movement was nurtured, shaped, and toned by Carl McIntire. We also have seen how he helped establish its major leaders and set the general direction of its ideological thrust. Further, by examining the history of his activities we have learned something of the history of the American Radical Right in this century. We have also seen the metamorphosis of Fundamentalism into a Radical Rightist political movement; and we have been brought up to date on McIntire's current activities. All that remains is a generalization concerning McIntire's immediate future.

Notwithstanding his current difficulties, Carl McIntire's immediate prospects seem to be reasonably bright. Even if his radio network is in some trouble, he was able to raise a 1970 and 1971 Christian offering of $1 million using this medium.[111] These were the greatest amounts he has ever collected; they exceed his 1959 offering by more than 1,000 percent. Moreover, since this offering is made up almost exclusively of small gifts, it can be interpreted as an indication that his following is either growing or stable. The total gross income of the "Reformation" movement in 1970 was, according to McIntire, $3 million, "more or less."[112] If this is correct, the organization's total income stayed at about the same level from 1964–71.[113] Reverses brought on by the FCC decision may have cut into this rather severely in subsequent years. But since McIntire's figures are his own and are unsubstantiated by any other source, the public Christmas offering is one of the best indicators of his power and general popularity.

McIntire's Cape Canaveral acquisition must be counted as his biggest coup to date, even though he may have overextended his organization. Generally, the trend of our times produces prodigious quantities of the kind of backlash and anxiety that McIntire has been able to tap in the past; and there is little reason to believe that the times or McIntire's skill will alter drastically in the near future.

7

Billy James Hargis' Christian Crusade

W hile the first chapter of this section concentrated on Carl McIntire and his "Reformation" movement, it also served to introduce Major Edgar C. Bundy, the Rev. Billy James Hargis and Dr. Fred Schwarz. The purpose of the remainder of this section is to concentrate more directly on these individuals and to develop relevant details about their movements. A few of the smaller Fundradist organizations will be briefly examined also.

Since considerable attention has already been directed at the centrally important ideological and historical details regarding McIntire and the emerging Fundradist movement, this portion will devote itself to comparatively contemporary details, and is meant to be more descriptive than interpretive or analytic.[1]

Launching the Christian Crusade

If there is any Fundradist leader who rivals Carl McIntire in power and popularity, it is Billy James Hargis of the Tulsa-based "Christian Echoes National Ministry, Inc."—better known as the "Christian Crusade."

Hargis' 1950 decision to launch a national crusade "for Christ and against Communism," his subsequent rise to national notoriety during the ICCC's "Bible Balloon Project," and the beginning of his radio network were recounted in the last chapter. It was also noted that, largely as a result of Hargis' concentration on race-related issues during the racially turbulent 1950s and his employment of the radio network and of a skillful public relations man, the Christan Crusade had grown quite rapidly.

In 1960 Hargis and his movement received another major boost. That year the U.S. Air Force distributed a manual which charged that the nation's "churches and educational institutions" had been infiltrated by Communists. It was learned that the author of the manual, a civilian employee, had used Hargis as one of his sources and had also recommended one of his ACCC pamphlets, "The National Council of Churches Indicts Itself on Fifty Counts of Treason to God and Country." The Air Force eventually withdrew the manual and issued an apology, but not before Hargis hit front pages and TV screens all over the country.[2]

By 1962 Hargis' "Crusade" was clearly one of the most important organizations in the newly formed Radical Right. At this point its annual income exceeded $750,000;[3] the radio network contained some sixty stations; an "international headquarters" was opened in Tulsa; an old resort hotel in Manitou Springs, Colorado, had been purchased, renamed "The Summit" and put into service as a center for various summer activities; the monthly *Christian Crusade* magazine was in publication along with the tabloid *Weekly Crusader;* and pamphlets,[4] tapes, record albums, and books were being produced by a sizable permanent staff.[5] By this time Hargis himself had obtained a B.A. and a B.D. (Bachelor of Divinity) from Burton College and Seminary in Manitou Springs, Colorado (Burton was identified as a "diploma mill" by the U.S. Department of Health, Education and Welfare in 1960). He was also awarded honorary doctorates by Belin Memorial University and Bob Jones University (Belin has also been classified by HEW as a "diploma mill," and in 1959, Dr. Clyde Belin, its founder, was sentenced to prison on six counts of mail fraud.) He had also met with South Korean President Syngman Rhee and

China's Generalissimo Chiang Kai-shek;[6] was speaking at as many as twenty meetings a month; had become an official Endorser of the John Birch Society; and had begun to take the lead in promoting unity and cooperation within the Radical Right.[7]

It should be noted that 1962 and 1963 were comparatively lean years for the "Crusade." For example, in 1961 Hargis had been broadcasting over two hundred radio stations in forty-six States and a dozen television outlets covering twenty States.[8] The reason for our choosing the year 1962 for a detailed look at Hargis' organization was because it minimized the risk of giving an inflated impression of the actual power of the "Crusade" during the early sixties. In retrospect it appears that Hargis had overreached himself in 1961.[9]

Hargis' "Crusade" began to regain its prosperity in 1964.[10] From a 1963 level of $677,200, its budget rose to $834,200. But in the meantime, the annual income of McIntire's "TCRH" had soared to the $3 million mark—making it clear that Hargis' "Crusade" had at least temporarily lost its position as the Fundradist movement's most affluent element.[11] Also, it is important to remember that since both groups depend mainly upon small contributions, their annual income is a rough measure of the size of their following. This reversal in income leadership is apparent in the 1958–65 figures (expressed in thousand-dollar units) for both organizations as well as for Schwarz's "Christian Anti-Communism Crusade," Bundy's "Church League of America," and the secular John Birch Society.[12] (See Table 1.)

Table 1
Annual income expressed in thousand-dollar units.

	1958	1959	1960	1961	1962	1963	1964	1965
tire	62.0	177.5	382.5	635.5	1163.0	1718.0	3000.0	3040.0
s	275.3	373.2	595.5	817.2	775.4	677.2	834.2	1106.9
rz	104.9	207.7	366.5	1209.0	725.5	573.8	616.5	604.0
	49.9	50.2	78.2	196.0	200.4	235.1	208.1	237.1
	—	129.8	198.7	595.9	826.1	1600.0	3200.0	4089.0

The statistics in Table 1 not only reveal Hargis' leadership and financial power during the early years of the Fundradist movement; they also show that it was not until 1964 that the John Birch Society became number one in terms of income. Since this was long after the contemporary Radical Right had become publicly prominent, it indicates that it was the Fundradist wing of this movement that furnished its initial impetus and viability. And during those crucial years, Billy James Hargis, even more than McIntire, was showing the way.

One factor in the "Crusade's" improved financial condition in 1964 was the passage of the Civil Rights Act. When this happened, Hargis' ability and predisposition to capitalize on racial turmoil paid off handsomely. But he now had to share the issue with the other Fundradists *and* the secular Radical Right as well. For they were all in agreement that this new development was un-American and, at least in good measure, Communist-inspired.[13]

Another development which generated support for the Radical Right in general and for Hargis in particular was the 1963 Supreme Court decision that outlawed prayer and Bible reading in the nation's public schools. Many Americans were horrified by this decision and the Radical Rightists were quick to seize the issue as still another example of "atheistic Communism" undermining the nation. Of course, this issue was tailor-made for the Fundradists and profitable as well.

McIntire immediately launched "Project America" in an attempt to generate nation wide support for a Constitutional Amendment to reestablish the outlawed practices.[14] Hargis also jumped on the issue, beginning a vigorous campaign that eventually led to active support of the Becker Amendment—a specific effort to amend the Constitution in the direction desired.

Just like Civil Rights, it attracted contributions and support from individuals who otherwise would never have become affiliated with one of these movements. Hargis' organization was low on funds and he pushed this issue especially hard—too hard in fact insofar as his tax-exempt status was concerned.

In late 1964 the Internal Revenue Service revoked the tax exempt status of the "Crusade" for its "political activities."[1]

Although these activities included such things as overzealous support of Senator Barry Goldwater's Presidential bid, the revocation centered on the "Crusade's" efforts on behalf of the Becker
Amendment.[16] Hargis thus became the first Fundradist leader
to lose his tax-exempt status. It was thought that many might
follow, but none did; and on August 9, 1971, Hargis proudly announced that his appeal of the revocation had been sustained by
the courts.[17] Moreover, a look at the financial record indicates
that, far from crippling his movement, the revocation may have
helped it by generating valuable publicity and by giving Hargis the
added isue of "liberal persecution."

Throughout the remainder of the 1960s, Hargis continued to
interpret the complicated and troubling happenings of the times
as the consequences of Communist subversion and neglect of the
Christian-American way. Race riots flared in ghettos throughout
the nation, a seemingly endless war ground on in Indo-china, the
nation's campuses were in turmoil, drug use spread from inner
city slums to suburbia, a counterculture emerged with hair brist-
ling and fingers extended in one or another sign directed at conventional society, and every one of these happenings served as an
auxiliary cause for Hargis' organization.

The rows of nameplates in the Crusade's new million-dollar
headquarters, completed in 1966, grew as the auxiliary causes
multiplied. By 1967 a staff of 70 and an 11,000-square-foot annex
were needed to handle the tasks of distributing the $35,000 stock
of books, tracts, pamphlets, motion picturse, filmstrips, tapes,
and record albums; coordinating the tours and seminars that multiplied each year; and operating the $35,000 mailing machine,
the letter writing machines, the signature machine, and the $27,000
worth of tape-duplicating equipment,[18] as well as all the other par-
aphernalia of an organization with a multi-million-dollar income.

There are some final comparisons and observations that should
be made. For example, unlike McIntire, who has consistently used
radio for fund raising, Hargis employs direct mail as his chief
means of raising cash.[19] He couples this with sales of tapes, record
albums, books, and other items previously described. He also
charges tuition for attendance at his "Anti-Communist Leader-

ship Schools" and for some of the other activities of his "teaching ministry." And all of these things are advertised on his radio and TV programs.[20]

Like McIntire's holdings, the extent of Hargis' radio network is difficult to determine. The figure for the number of stations has fluctuated wildly over the years. For example, in 1971 the *New York Times* quoted Hargis as claiming 70 stations.[21] For 1962, 1963, and 1964, Forster and Epstein give the number of stations as 200, 50, and 400, respectively.[22] *Newsweek* upped the 1964 figure to 500.[23] On January 23, 1966, Hargis told an interviewer for WTOP-TV, Washington, D.C., that he buys time on over 1,000 stations a week.[24] In 1967, Thayer mentions 270 stations in the network.[25] And in 1969, *Time* cites the figure of 100.[26] The 1970 figure was 115. This was furnished by Peter Schrag in *Harper's* after an interview with Hargis in 1970.[27] Hargis' associate, Gerald Pope, claims 100 for 1973.[28]

One thing this jumble of claims does suggest is that the number of Hargis' stations has, over the years, expanded as favorable auxiliary causes presented themselves, then contracted when the strength of these causes diminished. Further, there appears to be a hard core of approximately 100 stations that can weather all but the most severe contractions and provide the radio ministry with its major thrust. Surprisingly, the Federal Communications Commission does not maintain statistics on how many radio stations carry a particular program. The absence of these statistics probably encourages the Fundradists to inflate their station claims.

We have already described Hargis' use of "events of opportunity" to formulate auxiliary causes and enable his movement to prosper. The most outstanding example of the effectiveness of this technique is the sex education controversy of 1969–70. During this time the Hargis organization, led by its new "Educational Director"—an ex-McIntire employee, Dr. Gordon Drake—began a general attack on the NEA and the current state of public education. This culminated in an all-out assault on sex education. The attack struck a responsive nerve in many Americans and 25,000 new "Crusaders" joined the organization during just three months at the height of the campaign.[29] Soon the rest of the Radical Right followed Hargis' lead.

In 1970 Hargis claimed a total income for his "Crusade" of some three million dollars.[30] This represented an increase in one year of nearly a million dollars and, if true, it placed him about on a par with McIntire's "Reformation" for the first time in a decade. Since then he may well have eclipsed him. His staff increased to 104 employees and Hargis began collecting $452,700 in order to establish the "Crusade's" American Christian College.[31] He then began broadcasting in "living color" in a slickly packaged TV show. After peaking at 146 stations, Billy James Hargis and his All-American Kids settled down to a 40-station network.[32]

The American Christian College was functioning as planned in 1973 and Hargis' organization continued to operate smoothly. Hargis himself is casting about for new auxiliary causes and has been devoting most of his current efforts to trying to convince the nation that the United States is carrying out some sort of unilateral disarmament while the Soviets continue to build arms for world conquest and that the Watergate investigation is undermining the nation. But no single theme has yet emerged as dominant for this year.

Whether or not Hargis will be able to maintain parity with or supremacy over his old employer, Carl McIntire, is difficult to say. He has several advantages that may aid him in doing this. One is his youth. Hargis is not yet fifty, while McIntire is well into his sixties. Further, Hargis has been less troubled than McIntire with internal squabbles and defections. Finally there is some indication that McIntire may have overextended his organization in the Florida venture, while Hargis has been much more cautious with regard to organizational expansion. But Hargis is limited by his personal style, which is more distinctly regional than that of McIntire, and by his poor grammar and syntax, which must cut down on his appeal to the upper middle class. Yet, as is the case with McIntire, our troubled times provide Hargis with a host of auxiliary issues to choose from. And there is little reason to believe that he will choose all that badly in the near future.

8

The others

We have already learned something of how the Australian psychiatrist and lay Baptist minister, Dr. Fred C. Schwarz, turned from medical practice and part-time evangelism in his homeland to active "anti-Communist" crusading in the United States with help and encouragement from Carl McIntire and his followers. It will be recalled that two years after a highly successful two-month tour of America, Schwarz returned to stay in 1952, sharing radio time with the late Dr. William Pietsch of Waterloo, Iowa.

Not long after Schwarz's radio ministry began, the anti-Communist crusader told his listening audience:

> A group of Christian men have felt the need of alerting the nation to the perils of Communism. God has raised up Dr. Fred Schwarz from Sydney, Australia, as a special messenger on this vital subject. We are organizing the Christian Anti-Communism Crusade, a nonprofit Christian organization.[1]

After three years in Iowa, Dr. Schwarz moved his operation to

107

San Pedro, California. In 1958 he moved again, this time to nearby Long Beach, where his CACC is still headquartered.

From 1955 to 1957, Schwarz's organization scraped along on budgets of from $40,000 to $50,000 a year.[2] But in 1957, the Rev. Billy Graham arranged for Schwarz to talk to a group of congressmen about Communism. This led to his testimony as an expert on "International Communism (The Communist Mind)" before the House Committee on Un-American Activities.[3] This enhanced Schwarz's reputation considerably and provided him with his first truly national publicity. In 1958 the CACC's budget more than doubled to $104,900; then it doubled again in 1959 and more than doubled again in 1960.[4] These increases paralleled quite closely the fiscal fortunes of the remainder of the Radical Right.

The "Christian Anti-Communism Crusade" enjoyed its best financial year in 1961, one year after Schwarz's highly popular book, *You Can Trust the Communists (To Be Communists)*, came off the presses.[5] In that year—a bumper year for all of the Radical Right—the CACC's income of $1,209,000 exceeded that of either McIntire or Hargis.[6] Unlike either McIntire's "Reformation" or Hargis' "Crusade" however, Schwarz's CACC has declined steadily in income since then. In 1968, the last year for which data are currently available, the Schwarz organization's total gross was $464,274: less than half the 1961 level.[7]

However, these variations in financial success are the least of the differences between Schwarz, on the one hand, and Hargis and McIntire on the other. The most vital difference is that Schwarz is no longer a full-fledged member of the Fundamental Protestant Radical Right—if, indeed, he ever was. Even though he functioned as a lay Baptist preacher, put "Christian" in the title of his organization, and claimed that "God raised him up" to do battle with the Communist conspiracy, Schwarz will not currently acknowledge that he is either a conservative or a Fundamentalist. As Thayer says in *The Farther Shores of Politics,* "The only two adjectives he will acknowledge are "Christian" and "anti-Communist."[8]

This has not always been the case. When his organization was in its infancy, Schwarz spoke on McIntire's radio broadcasts, was

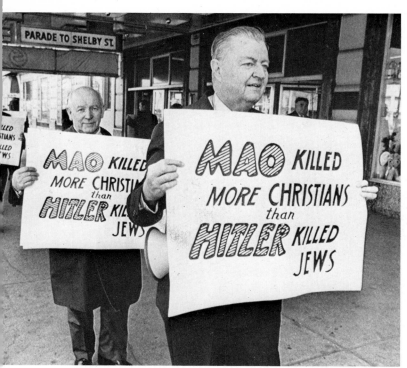

Carl McIntire (UPI Photo) leading a demonstration in Detroit outside the hotel where the Chinese table tennis delegation was staying.

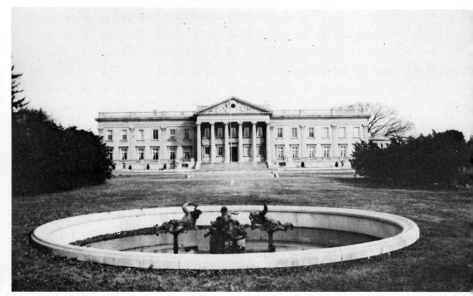

Carl McIntire's Faith Theological Seminary in Wilmington, Delaware.

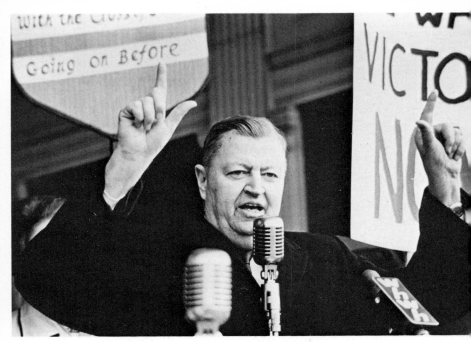

Carl McIntire (above) addressing "Win the War" rally in Trenton, N.J., winter 1970–71. Other people and posters (below right and top opposite page) from the same rally (photos by Ken Teruya).

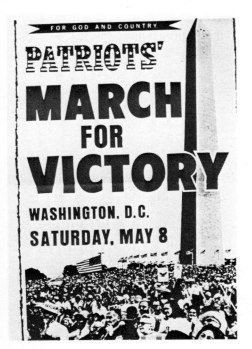

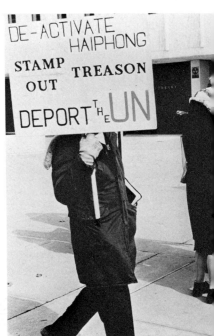

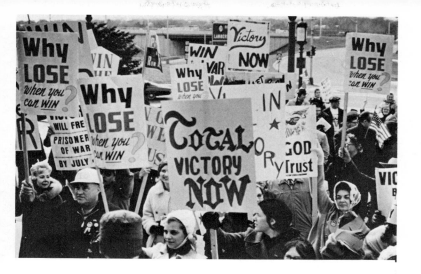

McIntire's floating radio station, "The Columbus" (UPI Photo), where he broadcast after the FCC shut down his former station due to alleged violations of the "fairness doctrine."

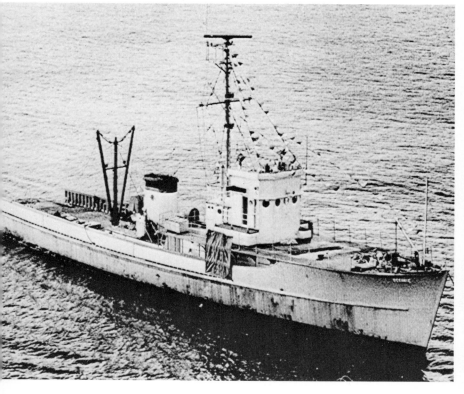

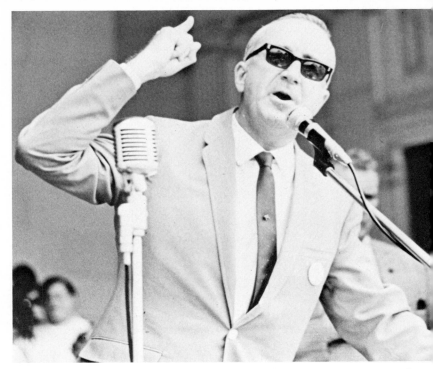

Major (Rev.) Edgar Bundy speaking in Trenton, N. J., at the 1969 rally and march protesting withdrawal of Shelton College's accreditation by the New Jersey Department of Higher Education. Below and on opposite page are more scenes from the same rally. The name Dungan refers to Dr. Ralph Dungan, Chancellor, Department of Higher Education.

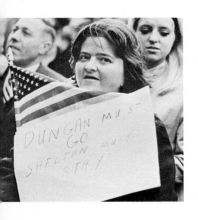

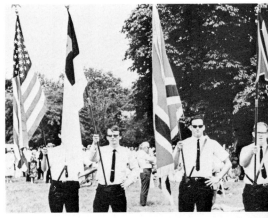

Four members of the National States' Rights par

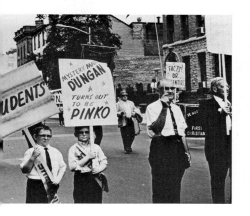
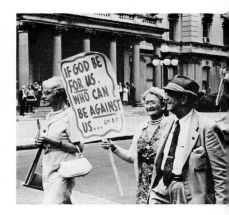

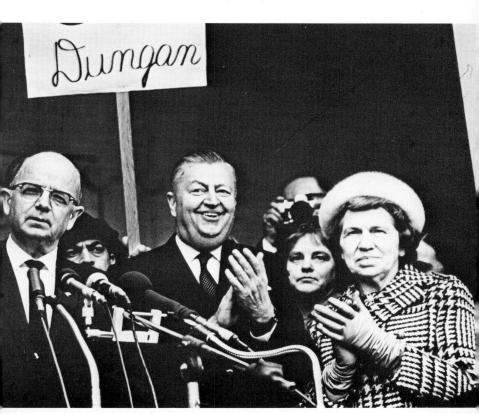

Governor Lester Maddox, Carl McIntire, McIntire's wife Fairy.

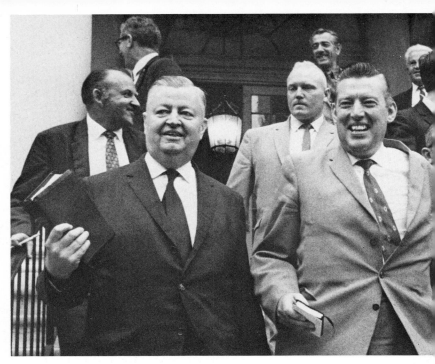

Carl McIntire and Northern Ireland's Protestant leader Rev. Ian Paisley (UPI Photo). Below is Sen. Joseph McCathy (UPI Photo).

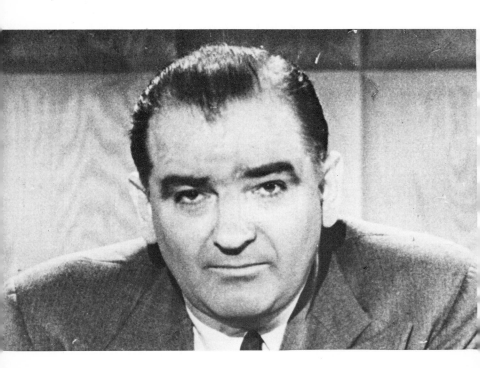

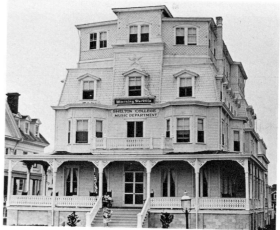

Cape May Bible Conference and Freedom Center's Morning Star Villa, formerly the music department of Shelton College.

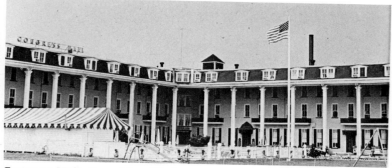

Congress Hall, Cape May, N. J.

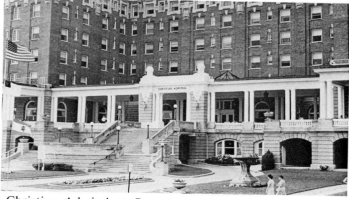

The Christian Admiral at Cape May. It serves as the nucleus of McIntire's Bible Conference and Freedom Center. McIntire broadcasts from the Top of the Cape Restaurant in this building.

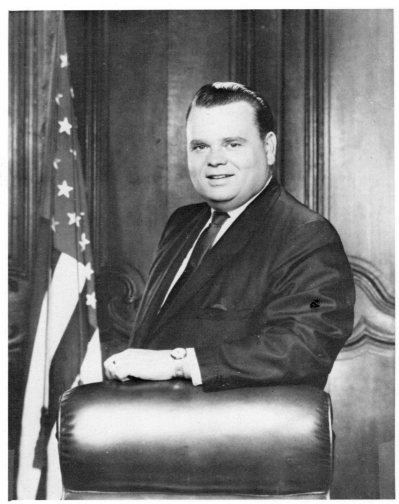

Rev. Billy James Hargis, head of the Christian Crusade (World Wide Photo).

an officer in the ICCC, and lectured at ACCC-affiliated churches.[9] In short, during this period he looked very much like a Fundradist in the making. But as his own "Crusade" got off the ground, a gradual change of direction became apparent. This change is succinctly summarized by Erling Jorstad in his excellent book *The Politics of Doomsday.*

> . . .Schwarz carefully moved away from any direct identifica-
> tion with the American or International Councils. He avoided
> any discussion of total separation; he made no direct appeal to
> Fundamentalists although he affirmed his loyalty to their basic
> doctrines; he made no overt connection between God's will and
> America as the Chosen Nation; and his premillenialism was ex-
> pressed in a highly muted tone. By 1964, he had moved more
> directly into the conservative camp, engaging Ivy League uni-
> versity professors for his conferences and associating with persons
> the ACCC-ICCC considered apostate; he had separated from the
> separationists.[10]

Schwarz also stopped the regular use of radio[11] and began to rely instead on his "Schools" of anti-Communism. Such schools are sponsored by local ad hoc committees, usually run for three days, require a "donation" for admittance, provide literature for a price, and are staffed by such speakers as ex-Congressman Walter Judd, Dr. Joseph Dunner of Yeshiva University, Dr. J. C. Bales (who also helps Billy James Hargis) of Harding College, and Herbert A. Philbrick of *I Was a Communist for the F.B.I.* fame. By way of example, such a school was held in June of 1970, in Washington, D.C., with almost 400 in attendance.[12]

Clearly, Schwarz's earlier, more histrionic "schools" had the effect of activating potential recruits for more extremist causes and movements.[13] But now that he and his organizations have gravi-tated toward the more moderate right, the "schools" will probably have a mixed effect, propelling some further to the right but pulling others into a more moderate position.

A final noteworthy difference between Schwarz and the Fun-dradists is that he is relatively open about his finances and he does not bombard his supporters with constant appeals for funds.[14] This stance is facilitated by the "donations" received and receipts for materials sold through his schools, as well as by his success in obtaining financial support from various tax-exempt organizations, certain businesses, and businessmen.[15]

Whether or not Schwarz's CACC is a Radical Rightist activity is problematic. Though Schwarz denies any such connection, Raymond Wolfinger, *et. al.,* recently summarized past judgments of the nature of his movement by stating, "Almost every social scientist or journalist who has described the Crusade considers it a radical-right organization."[16] This judgment is buttressed by Schwarz's past practices, including employment of acknowledged John Birchers and other well-known Radical Rightists as teachers in his "schools"; claims that criticism of the Crusade have a Communist origin; endorsement of the notion that Communist subversion pervades our society;[17] belief that we live in a dichotomous world at war, in which either good or evil must prevail; enthusiasm for "individualism" and laissez-faire capitalism; and advocacy of extreme methods to combat "Communism."[18] Furthermore, large numbers of his followers have held some or all of these views, and / or associations.[19] But all of this has been subject to the same slow but significant process of change that overtook Schwarz's position relative to the Fundradist movement.

Even though Schwarz and his movement are not Fundradists and may no longer even be fully qualified members of the Radical Right, they were examined for several reasons. First, when he began Schwarz was very much like the Fundradists if not actually one of them. But his later career demonstrates a movement toward moderation while McIntire and Hargis have moved in the opposite direction. Second, his movement's example brings home an absolutely vital point, *i.e.,* one cannot safely stereotype any segment of the right as either unidimensional or permanent, for Schwarz and his "Christian Anti-Communism Crusade" are neither.

Edgar C. Bundy's Church League of America

Currently Carl McIntire's "Twentieth Century Reformation" and Billy James Hargis' "Christian Crusade" dominate the Fundradist portion of the contemporary American Radical Right, Schwarz having drifted off to other ideological regions. But there is one other organization that is sufficiently important to be singled out for examination, Edgar C. Bundy's anomalous Church League of America.

We have already noted that the fifty-six-year-old Bundy served five years in the United States Air Force; that he was ordained as a Southern Baptist minister in 1942; that he later became City Editor of the Wheaton, Illinois, *Daily Journal;* that he was employed by Carl McIntire in 1949 as a combination public relations man and researcher; that he gained his first national publicity as an "expert" on Communism after testifying at a Senate Hearing; that he helped lead the ACCC-ICCC hunt for "Reds" in the clergy; and, finally, that he was appointed executive director of the Church League of America in 1956, launching his own career as the leader of a Fundradist organization.

The Church League of America was principally the creation of the late George Washington Robnett, a Chicago advertising executive. In 1930, Robnett began collecting the findings of various national and state legislative investigations regarding left-wing subversion in America. He also began accumulating a large library of publications that he regarded as "suspect."

Robnett became convinced that Communist subversion was a very real threat and that it was making particularly alarming progress in infiltrating American Protestantism. In 1937, with the help of Henry P. Crowell, President of Quaker Oats, and Frank J. Loesch, corporation lawyer and former head of the Chicago Crime Commision, Robnett organized the Chicago-based "National Laymen's Council of the Church League of America." The council's purpose was to "rekindle the spirit of valiant Christian Americanism" and to oppose "the challenge of destructive, organized radicalism." Its principal method was the dissemination of "intelligence data" to subscribers through its monthly publication, *News and Views.* The primary objective of the "League's" publication was to convince the nation's Protestant ministers of the reality of the Communist threat.

Robnett headed the tax-exempt "Church League" until Bundy's succession in 1956. During the last years of Robnett's leadership the "League's" budget had been averaging between $20,000 and $35,000 per year.[20]

When Bundy became executive director in 1956 the League moved its headquarters to Wheaton, Illinois. In this new location and under Bundy's leadership the League's annual income jumped to a record $38,500 the following year. The next year, 1958, it rose to $49,900.[21] In 1959 there was little growth. But in 1960 the League's income began climbing steadily—leveling off at the low-to-mid-$200,000 mark in the mid-sixties.[22] It probably has remained there since.[23]

Before the advent of Bundy's leadership the League had been sympathetic to the growing Fundradist movement, but it had remained relatively autonomous. Under Bundy's direction the League moved into closer alignment with Carl McIntire, establishing direct connections with the ACCC-ICCC and supporting virtually all of McIntire's activities. Bundy himself also frequently appeared at McIntire's side. But Bundy has never allowed the League to become directly affiliated with any other Radical Rightist movement,[24] even though he and his organization are in obvious agreement with most of them.

In the mid-1960s Bundy was conducting weekly fifteen-minute radio broadcasts over seventeen stations in eight states.[25] But by the summer of 1971 he had suspended all broadcasting,[26] probably because it was not paying off financially.

The suspension of broadcasting left the League with its major activities still intact. In terms of its size and uniqueness, the most important of these involves the collection, classification, and dissemination of "intelligence" data. It will be recalled that the League's founder, George Robnett, built the organization around his own collection of data on "internal subversion." Since then the files have grown enormously. Currently, the League claims an accumulation of over five tons of "countersubversive" data, including millions of cross-referenced file cards.[27] These are divided into categories such as outright Communists, sympathizers, and dupes. John Dewey, the famous American educator and philosopher, merits his own special section.[28] In addition, the League boasts of having an extensive library of "Leftist" publications.

The "intelligence data" derived from these files are disseminated in several different ways. First, the League publishes a monthly tabloid known as *News and Views* with a circulation of about 10,000.[29] This publication analyzes "current subversive activity" and serves as a major source of information on the activities of the Radical Right. It is supplemented by "Special Reports."[30] Second, anyone contributing ten dollars per annum to the League is entitled to request information on any four individuals or organizations, with each additional request costing five dollars.[31] Finally, Bundy himself lectures extensively and has written several books, including *Collectivism in the Churches* (1958), and *Apostles of Deceit* (1966), both of which were published by the League. Naturally, the "countersubversive" files furnish most of the raw materials for both the writing and lecturing activities.

Labeling individuals and / or groups as treasonous or dupes of traitors, without any due process or guarantee of elementary fairness, good judgment, or honesty, is unsettling to say the least. Yet this is precisely the primary business of the Church League of America. In fact, in the late 1960s Bundy attempted to push this type of activity even further. His organization sent solicitation letters to selected businessmen offering to "determine the philosophy of life" of any of their prospective employees. These letters stated in part:

> Our working forces include more than a few radicals, socialists, revolutionaries, communists and troublemakers of all sorts. The colleges and schools are educating and training thousands more who will be seeking employment.

The League's letter then offered to use its files "which are second only to the FBI" to ". . .supply you with all the data regarding your people that you deem advisable." Finally, the letter advised that the League was tax-exempt.[32]

This tactic apears to have succumbed to the exposés written by Mike Royko, a columnist for the Chicago *Daily News*.[33] But there is little to prevent its revival and eventual extension to school boards, superintendents, and principals in order that they might check on the "philosophy of life" of present or prospective professional staff—hardly a cheerful prospect.

Besides providing "intelligence data" for the Radical Right,

Bundy's Church League offers other services out of its $250,000 headquarters in Wheaton, Illinois. They include the usual run of filmstrips, tapes, movies, speeches, and books which have become the standard fare of virtually all Radical Rightist organizations. The only thing unusual about Bundy's activities is that they generally seem to supplement rather than duplicate the efforts of men like Hargis and McIntire.[34]

And this gives us a clue to the essential nature of Bundy's movement. It functions as a kind of support element—a rear-echelon back-up which helps bolster the front lines at thin points and provides much of the ammunition for the cause. Bundy is no McIntire. But he provides McIntire and, to a lesser extent, the other Fundradist leaders with a very valuable kind of support. In addition, he adds his own independent efforts to the promulgation of the ideology.

Others

It is difficult to determine where to draw the line regarding description of the various Fundradist leaders and their movement. There are, for example, certain movements that share many of the characteristics of the Fundradists yet are much more overtly anti-Semitic and / or racist. Gerald L. K. Smith's Christian Nationalist Crusade is one example. The Smith Crusade's last available income figure was almost $340,000 for 1966, indicating it is a considerable operation. But Smith's long connection with overt and virulent anti-Semitism[35] places him on or beyond the covertly racist fringe of the Fundradist movement.

Then there are those movement which share many characteristics with the Fundradists but which add an armed paramilitary element. Examples of this would include the closely connected Church of Jesus Christ—Christian, the paramilitary Christian Defense League, and the U.S. Rangers (sometimes known as the California Rangers). They share leaders and members, and the entire structure is overlaid with a quasi-Fundradist variety of Protestantism that also happens to be liberally laced with truly vitriolic racism.[36]

On still another level there are organizations that loosely connect Christianity with ultraconservative Americanism and laissez-faire capitalism, yet do not always adhere to an overtly Fundradist brand of theology. Howard Kershner's Christian Freedom Foundation—sporting a regular radio show, a syndicated column in over 700 papers, and a publication (*Christian Economics*) sent free to some 200,000 ministers—is an excellent example of this type of movement.[37]

Given the blurring that occurs on the fringes of the Fundradist movement, the major examples cited in this section were chosen either because they were clearly in the center of the Fundradist order of things or, as in the case of Schwarz, because they had some peculiarity or difference that was particularly illuminating.

There are others who, if space had permitted, could have been profitably examined. These include Dr. C. W. Burpo and his "Bible Institute of the Air." Burpo's major activity is his radio broadcast, which is carried by twenty-five to thirty stations in fifteen states.[38] He generally sticks to the Fundradist line, slightly modified for an older audience. His favorite ploy is to recount his personal physician's dire warning to "slow down" and then say that he has no choice but must forge ahead for God and country. Then there is the Rev. Dr. Bill Beeny of St. Louis, Missouri, who both broadcasts and travels his own lecture circuit. He generally adheres, in a decidedly rustic manner, to Fundradist doctrine and is primarily distinguished by his obvious lack of education and the curious items he sells to his followers. These include a tear gas gun that renders an attacker helpless and dyes him red for easy police identification and various "truth packs" which enable one to understand who really killed Bobby Kennedy or what cities are currently scheduled for a Communist takeover.[39] The Rev. Beeny has recently disappeared from the author's view.

Finally we should mention two individuals whose futures appear promising in the Fundradist scheme of things. The first is the Rev. Paul D. Lindstrom, pastor of the Church of Christian Liberty near Chicago and a primary organizer of the Remember the Pueblo Committee. In this latter capacity, Lindstrom garnered much valuable national publicity when he managed to be the first to an-

nounce that the crew had been freed.[40] Since then his activities have
been noted in *Newsweek* and the *Wall Street Journal*.[41] If he can
capitalize on this publicity he may go far.

The other man to watch is Dr. William S. McBirnie of Glendale,
California. Although McBirnie was listed in the *First National
Director of Rightist Groups* of 1963,[42] no mention was made of
his "Voice of Americanism" organization. It originated sometime
after his United Community Church of Glendale was organized
in 1961, but precisely when is not clear. McBirnie's "Voice of
Americanism" includes a daily radio program which started on the
West Coast and is now spreading elsewhere and a small publishing activity which specializes in McBirnie's own writings. These
include several vitriolic attacks on sex education. By the summer
of 1971 McBirnie had sixty stations in his radio network and the
rate of growth suggests that more may be coming. His theology
appears more flexible than that of Carl McIntire and this may give
him an advantage in the scramble for position which will inevitably
occur when the Rev. McIntire dies or retires.

Of course, there are literally hundreds of individuals, usually
pastors, scattered about the country who conduct activities which
are essentially Fundradist in nature. But there is little point for
present purpose in trying to pry them from the relative obscurity
in which they operate. Suffice it to say that their services are indi-
vidually small but collectively vital.

section 3

The Fundradist ideology

9

Fundamentalism

What is the world view of the Fundamental Protestant Radical
Right? What are their principal beliefs and how cohesive is
this belief system? How can they be distinguished from the more
general category of Fundamental Protestantism? In what ways are
they different from the rest of the Radical Right? These and related
questions will be dealt with in this section.

The difficulty in separating elements
of the Radical Right

While it is easy *in principle* to establish the distinction between
Fundradists and the remainder of the Radical Right, it is not as easy
in practice. This is because Fundradist organizations are arranged
on a continuum which ranges from Radical Right with no *overt*
Fundamental Protestant beliefs or attitudes to Fundamental Protestant with the suggestion of Radical Right propensities. As a
consequence of this distribution along a continuum, any attempt
to clearly distinguish Fundradists from the rest of the Radical
Right, or from groups bordering on the Radical Right, is subject
to some very basic limitations.

119

The problematic nature of the situation is further compounded by the fact that the continuum is multidimensional. Not only must the overt display of beliefs and attitudes be dealt with, but the matter of covert factors as well. For example, we may be confronted with a Radical Rightist organization which never overtly endorses any Fundamental Protestant theology. Yet, this organization might well be a secular offshoot of this very same theology. In other words, they could be "fundamentalist" in everything but their overt expression of opinion about theological matters.

Eric Hoffer speaks of the "true believers'" propensity for "religiofication." This is "the art of turning practical purposes into holy causes."[1] Richard Hofstadter argues that the world view of the entire Radical Right is essentially "theological" in character and deeply rooted in the nation's history of dogmatic, intolerant Protestant fundamentalism. He speaks of these groups having a "secularized fundamentalist mind."[2] These two views indicate just how untenable any hard and fast line between the Fundradists and the rest of the Radical Right would actually be.[3]

As a final comment on the difficulty of separating Fundradists from the remainder of the Radical Right, it should be noted that there is quite an interplay between them in terms of membership, speakers, "research," leadership, activities, and resources. They generally support one another's endeavors, at least in principle, and their mutual interdependence is often quite complex.

The John Birch Society

An example that serves to illustrate this observation is the relationship between the secular John Birch Society and some of the more well-known Fundradist leaders and movements. Since membership in the Birch Society is secret, there is no way of saying how many Fundradists actually belong. Nevertheless, there is considerable evidence that the relationship is generally quite cordial.

One indication of this cordiality is the presence of Fundradist literature in many of the Society's American Opinion Bookstores.[4] These stores specialize in disseminating the views of the Society as well as those of other right-wing writers.[5] It is not uncommon to discover materials written or sponsored by such well-known Fundradist leaders as Billy James Hargis, Carl McIntire, and Edgar C. Bundy on their shelves.[6]

Nor is there any absence of Birch Society literature, or works written by prominent Society members, from the activities of leading Fundradists. For example, Reformation Books of Collingswood, New Jersey, is a bookstore which specializes in disseminating the views of Carl McIntire. This store has a considerable amount of material available that was written by Society members.[7] Billy James Hargis has also been known to sell Society literature. For instance, it was available at his 1966 Anti-Communism Leadership School in Tulsa, Oklahoma.[8] This pattern tends to be followed by the remaining Fundradist organizations. Some of the smaller operators such as the Rev. Bill Beeny of St. Louis tend to use Society materials very extensively.[9]

If either American Opinion Bookstores, Reformation Books, or Hargis "schools" made it a point to offer the public a well-rounded selection of reading material the mere presence of each other's literature would establish nothing. However, the fact is that they all tend to stock only that material with which they are in basic agreement.[10]

Both McIntire and Hargis have expressed a positive opinion of the John Birch Society. The April 4, 1961, issue of the *San Francisco Chronicle* quotes Rev. McIntire as saying that the Society is "a good patriotic American organization."[11] Rev. Hargis is so enthusiastic that he is one of the Society's official Endorsers.[12] He has labeled Robert Welch, the Society's founder, as "a great American patriot."[13]

Hargis' relations with the Society go beyond endorsing it and its founder and disseminating their literature. Two Christian Crusade advisers are also members of the Birch Society Council, Tom Anderson and F. Gano Chance.[14] Hargis has produced a fifteen-minute color film starring John Rousselot, the Society's Public Relations Director since 1966,[15] and has also employed prominent Birchers as speakers at his crusades and as faculty members in his "Anti-Communist Leadership Schools."[16]

The interaction between the John Birch Society and the Fundradist movement could be worked out in much greater detail. How-ever, these preliminary observations are sufficient to illustrate just how closely their activities intertwine.

This is also true of the Fundradist relationship with the rest of the Radical Right. Throughout this segment of American society we find the aforementioned convoluted mixing of membership, speakers, "research," leadership, activities, and resources. All of this serves to warn the reader that in isolating the Fundradists in order to examine them, we are creating an artificial situation that is potentially misleading. These preliminary remarks are aimed at minimizing this potential.

Fundamentalist theology

Fundamentalism is largely a product of this century. Although its doctrines are deeply set in the soil of past centuries, its contem-porary thrust and name can be traced to a series of twelve pam-phlets, *The Fundamentals: A Testimony to the Truth,* which ap-peared in the years 1910 and 1912.[17] These pamphlets were a reaction to the spread of modernism. They dealt with subjects like the virgin birth of Christ, his physical resurrection, the literal infal-libility of the Bible, and the substitutionary blood atonement.

A group of conservative Protestant leaders adopted the term "Fundamental" from this series of pamphlets and set about to combat the spread of modernism. To this end the World's Christian Fundamentals Association was founded in 1918. Although the original movement was primarily Baptist in origin, it soon spread to other denominations.[18]

The Fundamentalists stood four square against any other inter-pretation of the Bible than that it was directly inspired by God and literally infallible. They bitterly resisted any use of modern historical research and criticism. They maintained that the Bible contained no myths and that it could only be interpreted as a series of statements of fact. They also opposed religious involve-ment in the achievement of social justice and declared the social gospel movement to be an apostasy.[19] (Apostasy is the abandon-ing of a faith.)

The movement's most marked characteristic was its predilection for opposing virtually every aspect of modern life. This negativism was not confined to theological matters. It became the last ditch position of rural and small-town Protestant America. It was here that the encroachments of cosmopolitan sophistication and its attendant rationalism were to be resisted to the end.[20]

Fundamentalism may have reached its apogee, in terms of its national influence, during the evolution controversy of the 1920s.[21] Nevertheless, it is currently attracting many new members. In fact, shorn of some of its dogmatism and self-righteousness by the abrasive effect of the twentieth century, the Fundamentalist movement contains some of the fastest growing church groups in the country.[22]

Fundradist theological pronouncements fall squarely in the center of old style Fundamentalism in its most dogmatic and intolerant form. While other Fundamentalist groups have shown signs of reaching some accommodation with the times, the Fundradists continue to resist, striking out at all who refuse to confirm their beliefs.

Although there is some variation, Fundradist theological doctrine is relatively homogeneous. The variation that does exist is due primarily to various levels of sophistication rather than any basic doctrinal differences. Briefly stated, this doctrine maintains that the Bible, in its original languages, is the literal word of God and is the only infallible rule of faith and practice. It maintains that Jesus Christ was the actual sinless son of God, that he was born of a virgin, that he died in substitutionary atonement for the sins of men, that he was resurrected from the dead still in his human form, and that he will come a second time in power and glory. The doctrine further maintains that man has been rendered sinful through Adam's fall and that his only hope of salvation lies in grace through faith and not in any worldly works. Finally, it proclaims that the saved will have everlasting life in Heaven while the lost will suffer unimaginably in the very real fires of Hell.[23]

This theological doctrine is a recapitulation of the traditional faith of many generations of American Protestants, and while this old literalism has been rejected by many, it still survives. It is the religion of simpler days, when preachers spoke of Hell as experts. It is the religion that died the death of a thousand compromises at the hands of the empirical tradition. But it lives on for those who are unaware of these compromises.[24]

It is also the religion of the Madison Avenue, computerized, 14-million-dollar-budgeted Billy Graham Evangelical Association. Far removed from the often humble physical circumstances of many Fundamentalist churches, Billy Graham still preaches a band of Gospel that is in close agreement with the Fundamentalist position. His status as friend of four presidents, and as one of the most popular and influential religious men in the nation indicates that a large number of Americans find such a creed to be at least plausible, if not the governing force in their lives.[25]

How then can we claim that the Fundradists are members of the Radical Right if their theological doctrine is so obviously acceptable to many Americans? The answer to this is simple. It is because this Fundamentalist theological doctrine incorporates only a portion, some would say a minor portion, of their ideology.

10

The political component

O ne of the most obvious indicators that the Fundradists are not just another variety of Protestant Fundamentalist is their tremendous emphasis on an intense "anti-Communism" as an essential part of their ideological stance. It is one of the basic commitments that binds the Fundradists together and marks them as a different breed.[1]

The vital importance of this "anti-Communist" belief element is illustrated by the fact that Fundradists not only characterize themselves as ministers of the Lord, but also as "leading anti-Communists." For example, Carl McIntire obviously sees himself in this way when he says, "Here I am, an anti-Communist, one of the strongest in the country and proud of it."[2] Billy James Hargis states, ". . .Christian Crusade is proud to be in the forefront of the eternal battle against Godless Communism."[3] And so it goes throughout the Fundradists in particular and the Radical Right in general. They are united in a common hatred of a very loosely defined "Communism." What distinguishes the Fundradist from the rest of the Radical Right is the way in which the "anti-Communist" ideological element is transferred from a political to a religious issue.

Fundradists see the fight against "Communism" as a holy crusade against a force that is the very embodiment of evil. Carl McIntire describes this crusade as ". . .the battle between God and anti-God, between God and the god state."[4] He describes the Devil as the "enemy of liberty" and "the author of tyranny and confusion. . .the one who is unquestionably deceiving the nations at the present time."[5] And he leaves no doubt that he views his loosely defined "Communism" as the chief agent of this Satanic threat.

Hargis also believes that the battle against "Communism" is basically a religious one. He describes it as ". . .Christ versus antiChrist, God versus Satan, light versus darkness. . ."[6] Hargis' "Christian Crusade" is directed against what he believe to be the ultimate embodiment of evil, international "Communism." The McIntire and Hargis statements concerning the importance of this "Communist" threat are typical of the Fundradist movement.

The Manichean dichotomy

Fundamentalists see the world divided between the saved and the damned and between good and evil.[7] Fundradists give this Manichean orientation an "anti-Communist" twist. The dividing line between them is sometimes indistinct. For example, in the early 1950s Billy Graham "strongly suspected that the spread of Communism was the work of Satan," and "he seriously considered leading a crusade against it."[8] That he did not do so is less important than the fact that such a course of action fits nicely into a Fundamentalist belief system.

Eric Hoffer argues that the "true believer" can exist without a belief in God, "but never without belief in a Devil." He further maintains that the strength of the mass movement arising from the "true belief" is "directly proportional to the vividness and tangibility of its Devil."[9]

Conspiracy theory

This Devil is made all the more vivid and tangible by associating it with a conspiratorial theory of history. Everywhere they see the plot, the hidden meaning. This conspiratorial theory is used to explain a world gone sour while under God's jurisdiction. Of course the current conspirators are the "Communists." And since Communism is a tool of the Devil it follows that the cunning, baseness, and diabolic nature of this conspiracy far surpasses normal human ability. Only Satan, working his will through the essential baseness of man, can account for the evil that is so obviously abroad in the land.

This "Communist" conspiracy is portrayed by Fundradists as most intense in its internal form. The termitelike burrowings of these agents of Satan are seen to be everywhere. They are in our schools, in the government, in the military, behind fluoridation, motivating the ecology drive, and most certainly in the modernist clergy. Over and over again the Fundradists emphasize this domestic threat that they perceive to be ubiquitous.[10]

David Noebel, an Associate Evangelist in Hargis' Christian Crusade, exemplifies this tendency. In his book, *Rhythm, Riots and Revolution,* which analyzes the way in which modern music is being used to "subvert" young Americans, Noebel claims, "The damage already done to this country through his [Pete Seeger's] influence is *impossible to calculate*." (p. 194). "It is our studied opinion that the Communists and the pro-Communists have an *unbelievable influence* in the folk realm *far greater than most would dare imagine*." (p. 156). "The Communists. . .have contrived an elaborate calculated and scientific technique directed at rendering a generation of American youth neurotic through nerve-jamming, mental deterioration and retardation." (p. 18). And, "The Communists are actually *molesting the minds of our children* through the *most cunning, diabolical conspiracy in the annals of human history*." (p. 156). (All the emphases mine.) This hyperbolic sampler could have been selected from any number of other Fundradist works.

ABSENCE OF AMBIGUITY. The concept of Communism as absolute evil contains no ambiguity, equivocation, or reservation. It is not just *an* evil factor, it is *the* very embodiment of evil itself. And it is not simply humanly clever. Communism's cunning is the cunning of Satan. Its plotting goes far beyond normal human ability. Only the power of God is capable of stopping it. And even then it will be a bloody struggle to the death, marked by no compromise and no quarter.[11] After all, you can hardly trust, or compromise with, the Devil.

Given this view of Communism, the Fundradists have no particular difficulty in dealing with the apparently contradictory evidence that it is now only a shadow of its formerly monolithic self. They believe that every time the "Communists" give evidence that denies the notion of their monolithic, all-pervasive, insidious power, they are actually demonstrating the unplumbed depths of their cunning. They take "three steps forward then two steps back." That is their dialectical method. Consequently, you cannot ever judge what they are after by what they are doing.[12]

Such a view is tremendously convenient. It allows the Fundradists to view the most damning refutations of their contentions with complete equanimity. All the contrary evidence is now just one of those "two steps back." Thus their view of "Communism" constitutes a "self-sealing" system. Every time the system is pierced by a bullet of contradictory evidence the sticky gunk of the conspiracy theory flows in to fill the hole.

STEREOTYPED POLARIZATION OF IN-GROUPS AND OUT-GROUPS. Earlier it was stated that the Fundradists' notion of "Communism" is very loosely defined. Perhaps because of their belief in the diabolical cunning of the enemy, they have a tendency to lump many separate individual groups and movements together under this general heading. Even those that are seemingly far removed from one another are all portrayed as belonging to this same category.[13]

Billy James Hargis claims that not only are Fascism, Nazism, and Communism "ideological bedfellows," he also claims that "a quick check of Webster's Dictionary will show that those systems are the same."[14] Carl McIntire asks if we are going to have "freedom" or ". . .are we turning to the left into socialism, collectivism, communism?"[15] After all, he has said that ". . .there is no essential difference between socialism and communism."[16] Hargis goes McIntire one better when he says, ". . .from this day forward, my friends, it (i.e., Christian Crusade) will equate liberalism and socialism with communism. . . ."[17] Frederick Schwarz has a more sophisticated approach than either of these gentlemen. He divides the left into Communists, Communist sympathizers, and pseudoliberals. The "pseudoliberals" are those who claim to abhor Communism but fight for the right of Communists to speak and organize. Schwarz claims that this makes them, ". . .the protectors and the runners of interference for the Communist conspirators."[18] And we all know that those who run interference are members of the same team as those who carry the ball.

This "lumping together" process is not confined to the area of socialism and Communism, nor to the extended area of liberalism. It is a general technique of the Fundradists and sometimes ends up with some surprising results. For example, McIntire seems to believe that "hippies" are somehow "Communists." On June 29, 1970, while conducting a radio broadcast over WXUR in Media, Pennsylvania, McIntire received a telephone call suggesting that he name one of his activities after Bernadette Devlin, the militant Catholic M. P. from Ulster. McIntire had previously labeled her a "mini-skirted Marxist." He responded to the call by saying, "Folks, we have the commies with us, the hippies." In another broadcast over the same station on August 6, 1970, McIntire "one-upped" himself. On that occasion he called the peace insignia a "Communist," "hippie," and "anti-Christ" symbol, all in the same sentence.

By lumping together all those who disagree with them under the general headings of "Communist" or "Communist dupe," the Fundradists succeed in virtually eliminating any middle ground. You are either *for* "freedom" or *against* it. You are either for *God* or for the *Devil*. It is as simple as that.

In such a black and white world politics ceases to be a process of compromise and successive approximation. It is converted into an either / or type of religious affair. It becomes a "politics of ultimates," where compromise is surrender and attempts at successive approximation suggest heresy.[19]

Creation of "social aphasia"

This "politics of ultimates" encourages a condition which theologian Franklin Littel has called "social aphasia"—a condition in which individuals are hampered or prevented from communicating

to others.[20] This is so because any attempt to communicate anything but agreement is interpreted as heresy, treason, or evidence
of personal gullibility. The Fundradists simply will *not* entertain
the possibility of their being wrong. A final example serves to
clarify this claim. On May 6, 1970, and individual phoned Mc-
Intire to take issue with him over McIntire's desire for military
victory in Vietnam. The call came during his air time over WXUR.
The arguments the young man used against the Vietnamese war
were of the same order as those advanced by several United States
Senators, as well as others of similar high and respectable status.
Yet when the young man finished, McIntire said, "A fellow who
is going to defend the Communist cause as you have, ought to be
dealt with." What McIntire meant by this was not clarified, but it
serves to indicate the way in which conscientious disagreement is
blocked.

Importance of chauvinistic religious nationalism

In addition to their absolute antipathy toward a very broadly
defined "Communism," the Fundradists share a proclivity for
chauvinistic nationalism. In modern times nationalism has often
supplanted religion as a focal point for fanatical belief.[21] In the
Fundradists we see a peculiar hybridization of the two.

It has already been mentioned that the Fundradists inject a
hefty dose of politics into their theology by defining "Communism" as an instrument of Satan. In addition to this, they define
the United States of America, at least in its mythic Christian-
American form, as an earthly agency for God. They view the nations. The loveliest of all home lands, and the most wonderful coun-
ment of virtue, God's chosen country.

America is described by Hargis as, ". . .one of the greatest gifts
that God has ever given man. . . ."[22] We are admonished to
"Choose Christ, for Christ loves America."[23] It is little wonder that
He does, for according to Hargis it is, "The freest of the free nations. The loveliest of all home lands, and the most wonderful country in world history."[24] Hargis believes that God has always had
elect people such as those of Israel and, later, Great Britain. Now
it is the United States that has this status.[25] Precisely how God ar-

rived at this selection Hargis does not make clear. Perhaps he was influenced by the knowledge that, "What civilization there is now in the world is due to the missionaries sent out from America."[26] It seems to follow that any nation so directly involved in doing God's work must have had His hands at work in her founding, and this is precisely what Hargis believes. He says, "America began as a Christian country, led by the Spirit of the living God."[27]

Such sacerdotal chauvinism is typical of the entire Fundradist movement. Carl McIntire describes God as the "author of liberty." He is convinced that this is where our ". . .concept of human freedom came from."[28] It was God whose ". . .thoughts are the ideology of freedom and democracy."[29] He inspired the founding of this nation.

McIntire depicts the founding fathers as Bible-believing Christians who ". . .accepted the testimony of the holy apostles and prophets and made their work 'the anchor of their freedom.' "[30] It was through the use of the Bible and the guidance of the Holy Spirit that these men were led to do what they did. He believes, for example, that the presence of the Holy Spirit was tied inseparably to their demands for political freedom. He maintains this because, "The best man who ever lived knows nothing about human liberty. It takes the deity to spell it out for us. . ."[31] And it is through the Holy Spirit that men are guided to do the deity's will. The fact that this folklore is at variance with the profoundly rationalistic nature of much of American revolutionary thought is simply ignored.

True to Fundradist form, McIntire, like Hargis, is capable of generating some truly astounding claims for America. For instance, ". . .it is our Christian nation that has given freedom to the world."[32] How he applies this to the American Indians or to the slaves owned by those Bible-believing founding fathers remains in doubt. McIntire does, however, give us some notion of the depth of Fundradist understanding of American history in talking about the issue of slavery. In his book *Author of Liberty,* he asks where the concept of human freedom, as contained in the Constitution, really came from. He then goes on to query "Why should it be wrong for one man to make a slave of another?"[33] The answer he gives is that it was God, through the Holy Spirit, who told the founding fathers these things. Apparently McIntire is unaware that the message must have gotten garbled. It was received by the founding fathers as three-fifths of a man.

This notion of America as God's elect, the vehicle of His will, distinguishes the Fundradist from the rest of the Radical Right. While both groups exhibit the characteristic of chauvinistic devotion to the United States, only the Fundradists account for the perceived superiority of this nation in this markedly theological way. For them, God and country begin to sound like one word.

The mythic America of the "Golden Age"

The chauvinistic patriotism that the Fundradists manifest is directed toward a mythic American society that they take to have existed sometime prior to the contaminating advent of non-WASP immigration and the hated New Deal. This mythic America of the Golden Age was the very embodiment of everything that Fundradists believe to be desirable. It was a place of full-blown individualism where every man was free of the constricting influence of "big government." In this America a man could use his personal initiative in the free enterprise system to seek his place in the sun. Competition separated the weak from the strong, and perhaps the chosen from the damned. The spectre of untempered ruin made sure that personal responsibility was preserved. The virtues of thrift, morality, religiosity, and patriotism held sway and men were handsomely rewarded for adhering to these values. People went to church, worked hard, respected their parents, took pride in the meanest jobs, gladly fought and died, and, most of all, were "free." All of this contentment, good order, and freedom were made possible by one thing and one thing alone. The America of the Golden Age was functioning in harmony with the will of God and the teachings of Jesus Christ. After all, as Carl McIntire says, "It is in His (Jesus') teachings and His deeds that liberty is defined, and it is these teachings that support our American system of freedom, private enterprise, individual initiative, personal responsibility, competition, and what we call the capitalistic system.[34]

An entire socioeconomic system thus becomes divine. To quote Rev. Hargis, "I am a Christian conservative today, because only conservatism in the United States espouses the philosophy of Christ."[35] ". . .Capitalism is the system that is in accord with Christianity. . . ."[36]

11

The pseudoconservatives

W hen the Fundradists call themselves conservatives and argue that they are simply trying to return America to her God-ordained path, they fail to present an accurate appraisal of their objectives and status. Anyone with an even rudimentary knowledge of American history cannot help but be aware that this America of the "Golden Age" is largely myth. Certainly, parts of that America had counterparts in reality. But for the most part it simply never happened. As a consequence, Fundradist advocacy of a return to this America is actually a plea to radically transform the present society into some kind of neo-Hebraic theocracy that has been fortified with a double shot of laissez-faire economics and nineteenth-century nationalism. Moreover, the delicate tension between freedom and order and individual versus collective needs, that is such an integral part of a democracy, lies buried beneath their specious reconciliation in a time that never was.

Devotion to a mythic "Golden Age" is no stranger to students of right-wing movements. It was a central feature of the ideology of Nazism and Fascism and is presently being emphasized by the right-wing governments of Greece and Spain, among others.[1]

135

Sacralization of the socioeconomic sphere

It should be noted that the entire socioeconomic sphere is sacralized by the Fundradists. As in politics, here too we have a system endorsed by God. Other systems loosely qualified as "collectivist" are antithetical to divine plans. As a consequence, advocacy of a socioeconomic system other than the one the Fundradists endorse is not just a disastrous mistake, it is morally reprehensible in the nth degree and actually heresy. In such a frame of reference McIntire's comments that ". . .the first and most serious charge that can be made against any form of collectivism is that it is idolatry,"[2] begins to make sense. The "politics of ultimates" has moved over to make room for the "economics of ultimates."

In their emphasis on economics as a determining factor in national life and values, the Fundradists find themselves in peculiar company. For it is precisely this same kind of economic determinism that dominates the Marxist world view.

The State as servant of God

Given their claim that politics and economics are essentially religious and that our particular system has been endorsed by God, how do the Fundradists deal with the Constitutional principle concerning the separation of church and state? Superficially they extol the virtues of such a separation. In fact, they often use this aspect of the Constitution extensively when they feel their activities are being hampered. However, their general response to this principle is bewilderingly circular. For example, McIntire argues that Jesus Christ is the author of the separation principle. He further maintains that it is ". . .absolutely essential for the preservation of individual freedom."[3] On the other hand, he says, "God is the one who made the laws for the liberty of His creatures and *the State must bow before them*."[4] (Emphasis mine.) And, "in the administration of the affairs of men, the State must be guided by the laws that God has made for man. Thus *the State literally* becomes a servant of God, and this is exactly what is taught in the Bible."[5] (Emphasis mine.) To dispel any doubt about his feelings on the matter, McIntire further states, "It is the task of the State *to minister as God would have it minister. That means that the standard of good in the judgment of the State, must be what God has ordained.*"[6] (Emphasis mine.)

Programmatic definition of freedom

Tying in the church-state issue with freedom and individuality, how can the "essential individual freedom" that Jesus is portrayed as desiring be preserved if the State becomes the vehicle through which Fundradist religious values are to be enforced? Furthermore, how can the Jesus-inspired separation principle hope to survive? McIntire solves these apparent dilemmas by closing the circle of his reasoning: "In ministering this standard of good. . ." the State accomplishes ". . .liberty." In fact, we are informed that there is an ". . .inseparable relation between Christianity and freedom."[7] This is so because, "When a man worships and serves the living God, he is free. When man bows down and worships and serves any other god, he is enslaved."[8] As Hargis says, ". . . there is no freedom without God. Where the Spirit of the Lord is, there is liberty. . .where the Spirit of the Lord is NOT there is NO liberty."[9]

Freedom cannot even be known without God: "Only when we start with the concept of freedom that there is in God can we have any idea as to what it really involves."[10] Every time man attempts to utilize this concept without God's guidance he ends up in ". . .all kinds of blind alleys."[11] For example, ". . .the concept of freedom offered in collectivism and controlled economy is man-conceived and ends in slavery."[12]

This programmatic definition of "freedom" runs through the Fundradist movement like threads in a rope and is profoundly revealing. Suddenly the right to be free becomes synonomous with the right to "worship and serve" what they define as God. Being unfree becomes, with a frightening simplicity, the act of believing something other than that which they believe. The implications of this concept of "freedom" do not require a vivid imagination.

Exercise of patriotism as a religious obligation

The reason for Fundradist nationalistic fervor is much clearer now. America, as a God-founded theocracy obligated to do His will, *demands* fervent patriotism as a religious obligation. God and the nation cannot be separated.[13] He is even inseparable from the intimate socioeconomic details of the nation's life-style. Consequently, as John Redekop states, "Since God and country are thus inseparable and constitute the greatest possible object of love and adoration, patriotism becomes another form of worship, and nationalistic fervor becomes evidence of true piety."[14]

All-purpose argumentum ad hominem

But this pietistic patriotism, it must be recalled, is directed at the mythic Christian-America of the "Golden Age." As a consequence, it is extremely useful as a tool to justify adamant opposition to all sorts of modern trends, such as civil rights legislation, open housing, unionism, the United Nations, the World and National Councils of Churches, and a host of similar matters. Functioning as a kind of all-purpose *argumentum ad hominem,* the God-given precedents of the "Golden Age" are the ideal instrument for the rationalization of nearly anything. If you oppose something, label it not of God and not of Christian-America. If you favor something, do the opposite. And since neither labor nor intellect is required to do this type of labeling, the most ignorant and / or lazy now need only to understand this litany in order to be superior to the most brilliant individuals of the culture.

For the Fundradist freedom, laissez-faire capitalism, traditional American values, political "conservatism", and "Christianity" are inseparable. Thus their "Christianity" comes to depend on other conditions. Without them it either cannot exist, or can only barely exist.

Departure from the religious mainstream

It is at this point that the Fundradists are most clearly distinguishable from the mainstream of Fundamentalism. The Fundradist contention that America is God's chosen country is viewed with deep misgivings by the majority of Fundamentalists. Some of them, such as the Jehovah's Witnesses, view any nationalistic devotion as idolatry and a violation of the universal nature of the Christian faith. Such Fundamentalists argue that Christ bore the meaning of history and that the United States of America is most certainly not necessary for or even essential to the carrying out of this meaning.

Edward Cain, in his *They'd Rather be Right,* demonstrates that the traditional Fundamentalist emphasis on faith as the primary criterion of religion is violated by the Fundradists through their intruding economic factors. It is no longer enough to "believe on the Lord Jesus Christ" in order to be saved. If you are a Fundradist you must also include the Christian-America of the "Golden Age."[15]

Of course there are also dramatic differences between the Fundradists and the non-Fundamental mainstream of of the Christian faith. In fact, with their emphasis on the Social Gospel, dialogue, Ecumenism, and human brotherhood, modern churchmen occupy a position that is practically antithetical to that of the Fundradists.

Franklin Littel, a well-known theologian of the non-Fundamental Protestant variety, illustrates the degree of division when he says that the Fundradists have "arisen in the midst of Christendom in decay, out of a culture-religion which has lost its eschatology and universalism. . .[They are]. . .in flight from the perils and anxieties of modern secularization, liberty, pluralism, and the challenge of the dialogue."[16]

Departure from the political mainstream

Just as Fundradist theology is far removed from modern Protestantism and even remote from much of Fundamentalism so their politics is at variance with past American practices. The already noted proclivities for destroying the middle ground, refusing to compromise, turning politics and economics into affairs of ultimates, advocating a theocratic state, and equating disagreement with treason, heresy, and gullibility indicate just how much they are in disagreement with these past practices. And there is still more evidence of this tendency.

Carl McIntire furnishes us with some when he talks about the type of devotion that he thinks should be directed toward his theocratic Christian-America. He says, "Nazism, fascism, communism, totalitarian orders are forms of idolatry. They demand allegiance and service from the people which should be given by the people to the one true and living God."[17] The full implications of this sentence require that it be savored. For it is in the implications that the flavor comes through. Apparently the major difference that McIntire perceives between various totalitarian systems and his recommendations for American is a difference based on the truth of the beliefs. He believes that the style or manner of commitment should be essentially the same. In fact, in other places he suggests that it is precisely the Communists' ability to induce widespread ideological commitment of the "true believer" variety that gives them the edge in the struggle.

This tendency to view Communism as a kind of negative mirror image of themselves is widespread among Fundradists. Time and again their various spokesmen express open admiration for the way in which the Communists are able to promote a sense of purpose and a spirit of unity, devotion, and self-sacrifice in their citizenry. In fact, imitation of the enemy is one of the most striking features of not only the Fundradists, but the entire Radical Right.[18] Consider, for example, the John Birch Society. It organizes itself into semi-secret cells, maintains closed membership lists, operates various "fronts," and in general pursues its ideological war in much the same manner as the Communists. J. Allen Broyles, in *The John Birch Society,* summarizes this tendency by stating, "One could define the functioning of the Birch Society in the same terms that Welch (the founder) uses to define communism. . . ."[19] It is in this area that the Fundradists and the rest of the Radical Right have one of their most striking and important similarities.

Earlier it was noted that the Fundradists are committed to the notion and individualism and concomitantly opposed to governmental control of economic institutions or interference with very broad-ranging property rights. While this is true as far as it goes, it fails to point out some essential facts.

Limitations of "individualism"

First of all, the type of "individualism" that the Fundradists favor is confined to the area of property rights and laissez-faire economics. Secondly, the major purpose of this "individualism" is that men may be free to serve God better, not that they may serve themselves better. This is illustrated by the fact that the individual is permitted no meaningful choice between competing socioeconomic systems. The choice has already been made—by God. It is for man to obey this choice. The same is true in the realms of religion, morals, and choice of life-style. There is only the way of God and the way of Satan. Individualism, in any broad sense of the meaning of this concept, is very difficult to fit into this structure.

Actually, the Fundradists' notion of "individualism" is strictly confined to certain narrow programmatic limits. These limits include opposition to governmental involvement in things like consumer legislation, social action to remedy social ills, medicare, unemployment compensation, compulsory social security, fluoridation, civil rights legislation, Fair Employment Practices laws and even antipollution measures. However, Fundradists do *not* object to curbs on individualism, governmental or otherwise, that are designed to force compliance with programs and standards that they favor. Rather they encourage curtailment of any deviation, however mundane, from that which they endorse, and urge that the government get deeply involved in such limiting activities. For example, they enthusiastically support Blue Laws, antigambling legislation, and other varieties of imposed "morality," and are at the forefront of those who demand that individual rights must be curtailed if the communist menace is to be stopped.

Absence of constructive proposals

Beyond their abstract opposition curbs on "individualism," in their narrow sense of the word, the Fundradists offer little in the way of policy proposals or plans that might correct economic or social inequities. Instead they offer a vague tomorrow when America might finally "wake up" and turn to their version of the Gospel of Jesus Christ. If this happens all inequities will simply disappear. Yet their Bible tells them that this arousal is unlikely.

And as if to support this message, they portray America as a place where gloom and evil are at every hand. Men, in massive numbers, are turning away from the God of their fathers. Drinking, card playing, modern dancing, nakedness, pride in the human intellect, moral relativism, collectivism, and, above all, the creeping red menace abound. There is only a handful of the real "Saints of God" left. Signs of the apocalpytic "end-time" are increasing at a frightening rate. And *all* of this is due to the fact that America has forsaken God's way. There is only one disease—sin. And there is only one cure—salvation through faith in Jesus Christ and a concomitant faith in Christian-America.

IMPORTANCE OF THE FALL FROM GRACE. It is at this point that the Fundradists' conception of man as fallen from grace through Adam's sin becomes vital to understanding this portion of their ideology. Their position is that, "There is no light in man; there is only death and darkness, tyranny and slavery."[20] Consequently, as Edgar Bundy states, "Sin is sin in any era; and sin is the root cause of *every* trouble in the world today as it was in 30 A.D."[21] (Emphasis mine.) And then several centuries of bitterly won knowledge concerning the profound influence of environment on man is waved away with, "Even environments do not change man's basic nature. Some (men) have had the finest, but they have committed scandalous crimes and violence on themselves and on others. Trying to change the world through economics, education, psychology and philosophy is hopeless."[22]

Now their "individualism" and opposition to "big government," "collectivism," and the "welfare state" is more easily understood. It is not that the Fundradists *necessarily* oppose the *goals* of many of these programs; though many actually do. Rather, it is over the *means* that the disagreement reaches a peak. Resorting to social welfare legislation in an attempt to solve social ills is not simply reprehensible. It is a sin against God, and it plays directly into the hands of the Devil. (The term "Commies" is virtually interchangeable here.) This is so because there is, according to Fundradists, only *one* solution to *all* of the woes of mankind. This solution, as previously stated, is salvation through faith alone. As McIntire states, "There is absolutely no hope whatsoever for us unless we return to the God of liberty."[23] Consequently, any other method used to solve social problems is evidence of heresy, and part of the fatal de-Christianizing of Christian-America.

All-important collective

Thus the Fundradists' insistence on what appears, at first glance, to be "individualism" is actually something less than that, or at least something other than that. It isn't the "individualism" that is so important, but adherence to God's law. In fact, when one considers the tremendous value that the Fundradists place on conforming to a certain religious style of life and on national unity, it is doubtful that their "individualism" even deserves that name.

In the Fundradists' world temporal ends and means virtually cease to exist. Everything is connected with the eternal and a God or Devil eternal at that.[24] As a consequence, if you advocate any position that is significantly different from what they believe it automatically becomes heresy, treason, or evidence of the grossest sort of stupidity. At the same time they see themselves and others in the world as Saints of God, Communists, Hippies, "Real Americans," Russians, etc. Thus they wrap purpose, worth, and destiny into the collective body. Outside of this collective all is void.[25] Where is the room for individualism here?

Denial of subjective good faith

It is difficult to imagine a more individualized aspect of human existence than a man's own thoughts. Nevertheless, the Fundradists are not even tolerant of any deviation in this area. Billy James

Hargis states, "If you THINK communist, you are a communist. If you THINK American, you are American and anti-communist. It's as simple as that."[26]

Arthur Koestler's *Darkness at Noon* captures the neo-Inquisitional and totalitarian quality of this type of thinking. One of his characters, speaking of the time after the successful Communist revolution, says, "We were compared to the Inquisition because, like them, we constantly felt in ourselves the whole weight of responsibility for the super-individual life to come. We resembled the great Inquisitors in that we persecuted the seed of evil not only in men's deeds, but in their thoughts. We admitted no private sphere, not even inside a man's skull."[27]

If we remember McIntire's suggestion that the man who objected to the Vietnamese war ". . .should be dealt with," it brings to mind that McIntire gave no consideration as to whether or not the man was subjectively in good faith when he dissented from the war. In other words, his subjective morality was of no consequence.

Subjective morality will not fit a world of black and white. As a consequence Fundradists are forced to brush it aside. And they are not the only ones who must do this. For example, in *Darkness at Noon,* Koestler's loyal Communist says, "For us the question of subjective good faith is of no interest. He who is wrong must pay. He who is right will be absolved."[28]

Denial of privacy

Finally, individualism cannot survive without the right of privacy and the right to be left alone, which Justice Brandeis described as the most important right of all. Nevertheless, the Fundradists, self-proclaimed champions of "individualism," honor the memory of that first Senator McCarthy and the era that he helped usher in. It is difficult to imagine when the right to be left alone and the right of privacy ever suffered more in America.

In order to illustrate the degree to which the Fundradists are unable to imagine the necessity for privacy and at the same time illustrate their fundamental lack of appreciation for the democratic heritage, one need only cite Edgar Bundy of the Church League of America. "No Fifth Amendment is necessary for those who are not afraid of the truth. They have nothing to hide, or of which to be ashamed. Their good fruit can be displayed without any apology or regrets."[29]

McIntire has his own programmatic definition for individualism just as he has for freedom. Speaking of the Ten Commandments he says, "It is the most individualistic charter that has ever been written. It is the eternal 'bill of rights.' It guarantees individualism. With it the individual is protected and preserved; without it the individual is crushed in numerous forms of tyranny."[30] Thus individualism, like freedom, now becomes connected with accepting the Fundradists' ideology.

World at war

Clearly, then, the Fundradists' endorsement of individualism is actually an endorsement of laissez-faire capitalism, except when it interferes with the almost unavoidable "war" to the death with Communism, or with certain convenient "property rights." The "ordinary usage" of the term, a social theory advocating the liberty, rights, or independent action of the individual, is inconvertibly out of place in the world of the Fundradist.

The Fundradists believe that war is inevitable if Communism is to be stopped. Surrender is the only alternative. What is more, the battle has already been joined. This "war" dominates their thinking. Even Fred Schwarz, who has disseminated a comparatively mild version of the Fundradists' ideology, leaves absolutely no doubt that he perceives the world in this manner. "The fundamental doctrine of Marxism, therefore, is that Russia and America are at war—not that they could be at war; not that they might be at war; not that they will be at war; but that they *are* at war. . . . *This is the frame of reference within which every action and thought must be assessed and judged.*"[31] (Emphasis mine.)

In a time of war, when the nation's very existence is on the

line, citizens must be ready to sacrifice themselves and their individuality for the sake of national unity if the war is to be won.[32]
Deviant behavior becomes tinged with treason and tolerance be-
speaks weakness and cowardice. Marching to the beat of a different
drummer becomes virtually impossible when the national drum is
beating out the rhythm of war. Yet this wartime world is the one
that the Fundradist spends his life in.

Leader principle

A society at war needs an exceptional leader. And Fundradists
are continually casting about for the charismatic figure that can
"wake up" the nation. This desire is reflected in the fact that
Fundradist groups are usually organized around loyalty to a single
individual. Carl McIntire and Billy James Hargis are both outstanding examples.

In the case of McIntire the leader principle occasionally reaches
heights which are truly remarkable. Clarence Laman was McIntire's
assistant pastor for some twenty years. In a booklet entitled
God Calls a Man (published by McIntire's organization in 1959),
Laman demonstrates these heights. He says, "Men, do you not
realize that Carl McIntire is our God-appointed leader? Who is
there among our brethren like him? There is not one of us to
carry on a work as he carries on."[33] Remove Dr. McIntire from
his place of leadership and you will see a disintegration of the
20th Century Reformation. . . ."[34] Laman then recounts several
examples of disruptive church members suddenly dropping dead
after questioning pastoral authority, one right in the church; then
he says, "It really has surprised me that God has not laid his hand
of judgment upon some who have been so persistent in justifying
themselves and making false accusations against Dr. McIntire."[35]
Lest the reader suspect that Rev. Laman could see no fault with
his leader we will cite his own disclaimer, "I am not saying Dr.
McIntire is perfect. Neither was Moses. But the accusations made
against Dr. McIntire will not stand before the counsels of God
any more than the complaints against Moses."[36] Rev. Laman was
replaced at his death with Rev. Charles Richter. He soon gained

the affectionate nickname "Amen Charley" for the fashion in which he responded to Carl McIntire's statements.

Demand for ruthlessness

It is in this wartime world that the moist side of the Fundradist rock becomes visible. Invoking the exceptional circumstances of war, they advocate exceptional means of defense.[37] One of these exceptional means is ruthlessness. After individualism is renounced for the sake of victory, kindness, charity, and "turning the other cheek" are not long in following. And, as Eric Hoffer says, "There is no telling to what extremes of cruelty and ruthlessness a man will go when he is freed from the fears, hesitations, doubts and the vague stirrings of decency that go with individual judgment."[38]

Sam Morris of San Antonio, Texas, ironically called the "Voice of Temperance" for his ongoing campaign against demon rum, was speaking on McIntire's radio program on July 9, 1970. He was speaking of what to do about modern day civil disorder when he said, "You asked me what I would do if I were President. I would do the same thing I would do if Castro landed paratroopers in this country. I would do the same thing I would do if the Chinese Communists landed paratroopers in this country. . . . Ladies and gentlemen, so far as I'm concerned if it takes troops and policemen armed with live ammunition to restore order that's what I would do. Let 'em have it with both barrels!"[39] At this point a member of the studio audience shouted, "Amen!"

Such open advocacy of ruthlessness and violence is frequently heard within the Fundradist movement. Rev. Bill Beeny, of the Gospel Revival Hour, Inc., furnishes another case in point. Speaking of Peter Fonda and other people who "criticize the country and make money doing it," Beeny said, "Why don't we get them all on a leaky boat for Russia and China; and if we don't get them all the way there, at least we will get them half of the way there."[40]

To the Fundradists "anti-Communism" is the central issue. The methods used by "anti-Communists" appear to be of little consequence, and the means are seldom regarded as threatening to corrupt the end. For example, in the summer of 1970 the Lutheran

World Federation canceled a scheduled meeting in Brazil because of considerable evidence that the Brazilian government was committing atrocities, such as torturing political prisoners, in order to stop what they described as "Communist-inspired" domestic strife. Hargis professed astonishment at such an action and said, "Surely they know that the Brazilian government is anti-communist. . . . I am so ashamed that the Lutheran World Federation has sided with the liberals and pro-communists against Brazil."[41] Among the other "anti-Communist" countries for which Hargis expresses admiration are Greece, Rhodesia, and the Union of South Africa.

Death of Christian love

What has happened to loving your neighbor as yourself, turning the other cheek, refusing to kill, and doing good to those that hate you? Perhaps they have become victims of the exceptional circumstances of war. But in any case, the Fundradists' advocacy of ruthlessness is not dampened by these Christian concepts. In fact, what they generally do with these concepts is either redefine them or place them in an extremely restricted context.

Hargis illustrates the redefining technique when he says,

> . . .Throughout the Scriptures we are taught that love is the keeping of the law. . . . And to keep God's law does not simply mean that you obey it, it means that you enforce it. . . . How do we show our love of God? By a silly sentimental affection for murders [sic] and thieves and killers and CONSPIRATORS? Heaven forbid. We show it by enforcement of God's law. That is love, and no man can exercise it without heroic effort. One must love God to punish a criminal just as a man must love his child in order to punish him."[42]

Any other form of love is impermissible in a wartime world. It would be interpreted as weakness or vacillation of purpose and could prove fatal. Or it could be used by the Communists as a smokescreen for their real purposes. Then, as Carl McIntire says, "Love is simply used as a weapon to destroy you."[43] Thus does love go the way of liberty and individualism, a casualty of the war.

Perhaps the ultimate in ruthlessness would be reached by those who would launch an atomic war. If this is so, then McIntire's particular group of Fundradists advocated a position that would qualify them for this dubious distinction. In 1948 the Annual Convention of the American Council of Christian Churches, founded by McIntire, issued the following statement, "For us to have the atomic bomb and, in the name of a false morality born of a perverted sense of self-respect and pacifist propaganda, to await the hour when Russia has her bombs to precipitate an atomic war, is the height of insanity and will, when the fateful hour comes, be a just punishment upon us."[44]

In the Fundradists' ruthless, intolerant, dichotomous world at war there is little room for those with grievances which tend to breach the absolutely essential national unity.

Role of racial bigotry

Championing "law 'n' order" and advocating self-sacrifice for the holy cause, the Fundradists denounce those who demand civil rights as "agitators" and suggest darkly that the Communists are behind it. In denouncing the civil rights movement in this manner the Fundradists simply refuse to look the racist nature of much of America full in the face. In fact, their resistance to any other solution but the spiritual salvation of the nation has led many observers to believe that overt racial bigotry is an integral part of their ideology.

This is a little too simple. While it is true that the vast majority of Fundradists are white, and it is also true that they often attract those who are vocally anti almost everything, they are not usually organized around racial bigotry as the White Citizen's Councils or the Ku Klux Klan are. In fact, some Fundradists, such as Carl McIntire, go out of their way to insist that they are not racially prejudiced.

Such denials do run into some very basic problems. Even if the leadership of the movement is not racist, the nature of the ideology provides perfect cover for those who are guilty of virulent bigotry but desire to conceal it, from themselves or from others. After all, it is much less troubling for many individuals if they are for states' rights, freedom of choice, or property rights, than if they are forced to admit that they just hate "niggers."

Overt expressions of racial bigotry, where appearing at all in the Fundradist movement, are generally found in the utterances of underlings rather than in those of the leader. Billy James Hargis and his Crusade furnish a typical example. Although Hargis himself once wrote a pamphlet extolling segregation as "God-ordained," and still proudly defends Rhodesia and South Africa as bastions of Christian freedom, he is careful to stay away from remarks that reveal naked bigotry. This has not been true of many close to him. For instance, General Richard Moran, Chairman of the Christian Crusade's advisory board, speaking at the 1966 Anti-Communist Leadership School at Tulsa, denounced the UN Charter as an attempt to create a ". . .Universal Brown man—the man with no race, the neuter man. . . ."[45]

The 1962 version of this "School" had even more overt displays of racial prejudice. At this time, Dr. Revilo Oliver denounced liberals for taxing Americans to death for the benefit of every "mangy cannibal in Africa"; and R. Carter Pittman claimed that the Negro race was biologically and intellectually inferior. He also maintained that the major differences between American Negroes and Negroes in the Congo was that "in the Congo they eat more people than they do in the United States." And all of this took place after Hargis cautioned that he would not tolerate intemperate statements.[46]

It should be reiterated, however, that this type of overt bigotry, while not difficult to find, is not typical of all Fundradists and certainly is not typical of the top leadership. Of course, the further south the organization, the more overt the antiblack feeling. But, in general, even then it is covert, usually disguised as something else, and commonly expressed in "code." Therefore, it seems reasonable to conclude that racism is not essential to the Fundradists' ideology, but is often found as a concomitant feature.

The same thing can be said about the leadership of other forms of bigotry to the Fundradist ideology. Anti-Semitism can furnish us one example, anti-Catholicism another.

ROLE OF ANTI-SEMITISM. In the case of anti-Semitism we have Hargis' General Moran again. It is his opinion not only that the United Nations charter is a cover for miscegenation, but that it is also an instrument created by the Rothschilds in order that they might control the world.[47] There is also Hargis' relationship to the Rev. Gerald B. Winrod, an individual described by the Anti-Defamation League of B'Nai B'rith as "a propagandist so notorious for his pro-Nazism and anti-Semitism in the 1930s and 1940s that he became known as the Jayhawk Nazi."[48] He helped Hargis establish his Christian Crusade. Then there is Allen Zoll, formerly on the staff of the Crusade, described by the ADL as "a notorious anti-Semite."[49] And so it goes throughout much of the Fundradist movement. Like anti-Negro sentiment, anti-Semitism is greater in some segments of the movement than in others, and greater in the underlings than in those at the top. It is at home in the 100-percent ideology of the Fundradists.

ROLE OF ANTI-CATHOLICISM. In the case of anti-Catholicism we have the Rev. Carl McIntire himself. McIntire vigorously denies being anti-Catholic. He may well believe this. Nevertheless, he has said,

> The strengthening of the Roman Catholic Church throughout the world only involves the fostering of a false religion which enslaves the human soul in darkness and superstition. . . . Rome will sell her secret confessional system for political world power. But actually the Roman Cathoic Church becomes a spy system through the priests, with the priests' loyalty first to the Vatican. . . . Are not Roman Catholics in the United States committed to a foreign power and do they not owe obedience and submission to its head, the Pope?[50]

McIntire has also brought the Northern Irish anti-Catholic extremist Rev. Ian Paisley to this country on several occasions. He has also returned these visits. Once he did so when Paisley was in jail for his activities. McIntire lauds Paisley as a "man of God" who has been raised up by Him in Ulster's "hour of decision." He even claims that there is no discrimination against Catholics in Ulster.

Given this kind of background it is little wonder that the Democrats labeled McIntire one of the five "major anti-Catholic extremists" operating during John Kennedy's campaign for the presidency.[51] And this is not all that can be said about McIntire's attitudes toward Catholicism, or about the anti-Catholic nature of some of his associates. Suffice it to say that if Carl McIntire is not anti-Catholic, then he is most certainly misunderstood. Nevertheless, the majority of his public utterances are not overtly anti-Catholic. And recently they have become even less so. And when, for example, one of his listeners calls while he is on the air, and expresses notions about the Papist plots or some such, McIntire is quick to redirect the conversation.

Submergence of overt bigotry

The important point to remember from all this discussion of anti-Semitic, anti-black, and anti-Catholic prejudice is that it is not *necessary* to harbor any of these biases in order to be a Fundradist. To be sure, bigotry and prejudice can be seen as related to the basic nature of this belief system. And it is true that if a person is Fundradist he is likely to be bigoted. Nevertheless, overt displays of bigotry, at least of the intra-American variety, are not usually encouraged. In fact, if such bigotry is to be expressed at all it almost invariably must be confined to some kind of anti-Communist format. In order to be a Fundradist your bigotry must be capable of being at least partially submerged in this other system of values. If such an observation seems a "splitting of hairs," one need only recall the existence of the K.K.K., the American Nazi Party, the National States' Rights Party, and similar groups. They know no such distinction. On the other hand, the line should be thought of as definite, for it is not always so. There are cases where the two blend imperceptibly.

A cautionary note

This is the ideology of the Fundamental Protestant Radical Right. But the caution offered at the beginning still stands. This group is not totally homogeneous. As a conseqcence, any attempt at capturing their ideological position is bound to be less than 100 percent successful. Nevertheless, the central flavor is here. And it is the flavor of a world gone sour.

Faced with a world become staggeringly complex, surrounded by the bloated bodies of multiplied sacred cows, some Americans were forced into a desperate search for an explanation of this trend. But not just any explanation would do. It had to be one which kept God on his throne and which retained for America a manifest destiny, for these were the things that they desperately wanted to believe in. Yet how could they, with all of these terrible changes abounding?

The required explanation, for some, centered on "conspiratorial Communism." Draped out in horns and tail and forced under the dichotomous rubric of Fundamentalism, this force could serve as an explanation for the changes while allowing belief in both God and country to survive. Here, at last, was the diabolical power capable of beguiling and betraying in the face of God's omniscience and the nation's destiny. And with this answer, the world became simple again.

section 4

Toward a deeper understanding

It has been demonstrated that the Fundradist ideology takes the form of an interlocking, convoluted complex of characteristics that defies simple description. Nevertheless, it did prove possible to isolate the ideology's most salient elements. These were found to be:

1. Fundamentalist theological beliefs in the verbal inspiration of the Bible, Jesus' virgin birth, his substitutionary blood atonement for a mankind fallen through original sin, his bodily resurrecton, his premillennial second coming, and salvation through faith rather than works.

2. A chauvinistic devotion to a theocratic "Christian-America" of the mythic "Golden Age."

3. An intense, albeit very broadly defined, "anti-Communism."

4. A conspiratorial view of history.

5. An almost totally dichotomous world view.

6. A dogmatic thought pattern reinforced by a predisposition for circular reasoning.

7. A resistance to most aspects of modern life.

8. A tendency to sacralize almost everything.

9. A relentless demand for conformity to their norms while simultaneously advocating "individualism."

10. A belief that the world is at war, a war to the death, accompanied by a desire for the employment of ruthless measures in order to win this war.

11. An opposition to any social reform not based on salvation.

But we have yet to examine any of the many theories that have been advanced to explain this ideology, nor have we attempted to place it in any historical context.

Without some background in both these areas our understanding of the ideology becomes a thread detached from texture—an intellectual raveling, if you will—and loses much of its usefulness. Thus the task of inquiring into the theoretical and historical roots of our subject is vital.

The most obvious way of doing this would be to separate this part of the inquiry into a chapter on theory and a chapter on history. A less severe alternative would be to give them clearly separate treatment within the same chapter. But either approach presents difficulties.

Much historical writing concerning the Radical Right has leaned heavily on various theoretical explanations of this kind of movement, the theory furnishing the historian a structure upon which he can arrange his facts. For example, Richard Hofstadter's excellent inquiries into the history of right-wing extremism in America made extensive use of a subtle and complex combination of such theoretical rubrics.[1]

Careful analysis of historical events is also capable of generating positions. In fact, a considerable amount of theorizing on right-wing extremism has had just such a genesis.[2] Thus theory not only provides a structure for the historian's use, it is also generated by historical analysis.

Obviously, then, theory and history interact in a complex fashion. And this is especially true when we are talking about the history and theory of the Radical Right. This particular segment of the American populace has captured the attention of the social sciences as few others have. As a result, there is a wealth of sociological, social-psychological and psychological theories and observations about them. And each one of these theories, or any combination thereof, is capable of providing historians with new directions. Indeed, a good deal of the most productive history concerning the Radical Right has been written with precisely that kind of impetus. And, as we would expect, historical research has also aided the development of theory about the Right. Thus, separating history and theory when dealing with this subject is even less desirable than would ordinarily be the case.

As a matter of fact, cross-fertilization has been so complete in a number of cases that any attempt to separate theory from history would result in the destruction of the entire position.

As a consequence of these considerations this section has been arranged in a mixed fashion. For the sake of organizational convenience it begins with a chapter on history and ends with one on theory. However, the theory chapter does seek to demonstrate the application of the theory to the work of the historian. Due to space limitations it was not possible to do this in every instance, but it was applied where the theoreticians themselves had done so. Hopefully this will be sufficient to demonstrate the interplay between theoretical and historical work and simultaneously enrich the later historical account by providing the reader with several alternative interpretations.

No attempt has been made to adopt any one of these theories as the basis for the historical chapter. But neither is this portion meant to be theory-free. Rather, it is deliberately eclectic. That is to say, it contains the results of picking and choosing among the theoretical alternatives in order to generate the most adequate description that the author is capable of. But one can never be sure that some theoretical bias has not crept in. Nor is there any assurance that the important contributions of one or another theory are not inadvertently ignored.

This brings us to the last, and possibly most important reason for combining history and theory in the same section: it serves to maximize the reader's ability to identify such biases or add the missing insights. In short, combination helps destroy the protective cover which hides mistakes.

The theoretical context

Status anxiety theory

T here is a general body of theory that attempts to explain the
contemporary Radical Right in terms of variations on a status
anxiety theme. This theme proposes that Radical Rightist politics
are a consequence of the projection of social status anxieties into
political movements.

Probably the richest single source of this status anxiety theory is
The Radical Right, edited by Daniel Bell. In this volume individuals such as Richard Hofstadter, Peter Viereck, Daniel Bell, David
Riesman, Nathan Glazer, Seymour Lipset, and Talcott Parsons
work out their own variations on this theoretical base. And even
though all of them built their position around this common theme,
the breadth of viewpoint and emphasis available in this one volume
is considerable. Thus we are reminded that any basic theoretical
position is open to dozens of significantly different permutations,
and each of these has its own historical implications.

Because of the unusual breadth of status anxiety theory and the
detailed historiography that has been done under its theoretical
guidance, three separate examples of status anxiety-based analyses
of the historical antecedents of the current Radical Right will be

reviewed. They include the work of three social scientists, Seymour Lipset, the David Riesman–Nathan Glazer team, and the historian Richard Hofstadter. These examples were not chosen because they represent the opposite polarities of status anxiety theory. Rather, they were picked because they are among the most popular versions of this theoretical position, and because they afford an excellent opportunity to illustrate the effects that differences of style and emphasis can have, even when the authors are in substantial theoretical agreement.

Lipset's variation

Seymour Lipset argues that during periods of prosperity there are numerous individuals who manage to obtain higher social positions. In time groups of these people form coalitions whose function it is to defend these newly acquired positions. Though these groups, formed on the basis of what Lipset calls "status politics," are not homogeneous, they are prone to generate a "Radical Right"[1] when their defensive action become extreme and pass beyond the normal boundaries of American politics.[2]

Using his "status politics" theory as a criterion for selecting the relevantly similar in history, Lipset cites what he claims are four examples of this theory in action. These are: the Know-Nothing movement of the first half of the 1850s, the American Protective Association of the 1880s and 1890s, the Progressive movement of the period 1900 to 1910, and the Fundamentalism of the 1920s, as exemplified by the Ku Klux Klan.[3]

He notes that each of these movements emerged during prosperous times and that its decline was marked by a decline in prosperity.[4] The one exception that he acknowledges is the decline of the Klan. This was already well along by 1926, even though the prosperity of the twenties lasted for two more years Lipset attributes this to the exposure of Klan leaders as corrupt charlatans and to the fact that the press and the upper class had subjected them to extreme social pressure resulting in the Klan's loss of respectability.[5]

Although he does not say so directly, Lipset suggests that the

Know-Nothings may have had their origins in the emergence of popular democracy during the Jacksonian period. During this time the "common man" won a new position in American society. By the the 1850s it was clear that his position was being threatened by the arrival of large numbers of immigrants, who, not so incidentally, were chiefly of the Roman Catholic faith. Know-Nothingism, says Lipset, was one consequence of this threat. And in this theoretical context it is small wonder that it took a nativist, anti-Catholic form.[6]

Lipset does not go into detail on the American Protective Association. In general he suggests that its anti-immigrant and anti-Catholic nature marked it as "latter-day Know-Nothingism."[7] Most importantly he argues that the movement was based on the same type of status anxiety.

Lipset's most interesting historical example is the Progressive movement which reached its peak in the years 1900 to 1910. This movement differed considerably from the others in that it was based on a desire to institute liberal social reforms. Nevertheless Lipset argues that it could very well have had its base in the very same kind of "status politics." Lipset cites Hofstadter's contention, in *The Age of Reform,* that Progressivism was based in large measure on the reaction of middle-class Protestants to threats on their social position.[8]

These threats came from two widely different directions. One emanated from the great millionaires of the latter nineteenth and the early twentieth centuries. They had taken over much of the influence that the older middle class had preciously enjoyed and threatened this middle class with the very real possibility of still greater loss of status in the future. The other threat to the middle class's status was the perennial favorite of those with status anxiety, the immigrants. For the immigrants and their children were gaining power and with it the ability to push America along a pluralistic road.[9] In concert, both of these threats were sufficient to generate, claims Lipset, the "status politics" that was called Progressivism.

Lipset's final example, the Ku Klux Klan of the 1920s, coincides with that of Hofstadter recounted earlier. He describes the Klan of this period as based on the anxiety of small-town Protestant working clases over the ever-increasing influences of "cosmopolitanism."[10] And, although he does not say so, it seems reasonable to think that Lipset's "cosmopolitanism" is very much like Hofstadter's "rationalism" and "modernism."

In what sense the small-town Protestant working class had "recently arrived" Lipset does not make clear. And this lack of clarity is important, for one of his major points is that it is the status insecurity of the newly arrived that generates the crucial anxiety. Whether this is simply an oversight or actually reveals a flaw of some importance is difficult to ascertain. Suffice it to say that it is a significant omission.

Riesman and Glazer's variation

David Riesman and Nathan Glazer, both social scientists, have their own version of this theory. In their joint paper, "Intellectuals and the Discontented Classes," Riesman and Glazer argue that it is the "new middle class" that is arising from urban working class neighborhoods and the "marginal small towns" that is the unique breeding ground for the contemporary Radical Right.[11]

They call this new middle class "the discontented." They theorize that it was out of discontent that the Radical Right grew. Part of the discontent is rooted in this class's relative economic deprivation. For they soon find out that the salaries they eagerly anticipated in their working class days do not go nearly as far as they had expected. Further, their previous experiences with very limited incomes have left them with a "pinched and narrow" type of fiscal conservatism.[12]

More importantly, however, the discontent arises from the necessity of having an opinion, now that they are middle-class, and of coping with the nation and the world as well as with their jobs and immediate surroundings. But the explanations available to them are disconcerting, dissatisfying, and even threatening. As a consequence many seek the simple answer available in the rightist brand of political extremism.[13]

At first glance it seems that Riesman and Glazer simply applied Lipset's historical-sociological analysis to more contemporary times. One is even tempted to claim that their position simply brings Lipset up to date. But such an interpretation could be misleading. This is due to the fact that the Riesman–Glazer position puts a heavy emphasis on the unique circumstances surrounding the emergence of the contemporary Radical Right. According to Riesman and Glazer the rise to higher status need not coincide with a period of general prosperity, a chief claim made by Lipset, nor will just any sort of upward mobility suffice. They claim that it must be upward mobility into the middle class and that general prosperity is not required. This is not to say that Riesman and Glazer reject the relevance of Lipset's historical parallels. But their position adds a significant new dimension to the search for relevantly similar antecedents of the contemporary American Radical Right. It does this by broadening the historical periods that must be attended to and by narrowing the human focus. The first of these is accomplished by eliminating Lipset's criterion, a period of general prosperity. The second is accomplished by including only those groups or individuals who have recently been upwardly mobile into the middle class.

Thus, for example, Riesman–Glazer would not balk at examining right-wing activities during the Great Depression for clues to the origin and nature of the contemporary Radical Right, provided they involved a significant number of individuals who had recently attained middle-class status. Lipset, on the other hand, would have to ignore these groups if he were to remain loyal to his own theoretical base. Obviously the Great Depression was anything but a period of general prosperity.

Hofstadter's variation

Probably the most well-known example of status anxiety theory that involves the contemporary American Radical Right can be found in Richard Hofstadter's 1964 Pulitzer Prize-winning book, *Anti-Intellectualism in American Life*. Like Lipset and Riesman–Glazer, Hofstadter is heavily indebted to this theoretical position. Unlike them, however, he develops this theory in the brilliantly descriptive fashion for which he was noted.

Hofstadter argues that after the Civil War the generally evangelistic American Protestant movement was forced to turn its attention from the prewar assault on religious indifference to the ever-growing influence of rationalism. This rationalism was based on Darwinism, heightened by a disturbing movement toward modern scholarly Biblical criticism that was emanating from the European continent.[14]

Hofstadter characterizes this post–Civil War period as one of increasing defection from the traditional religious position. Ministers and laymen alike, many with evangelical beliefs, found themselves swayed by these rationalistic influences. And more and more of them turned to the emerging modernist church.[15]

Those who did not found themselves becoming increasingly isolated. Moreover they were losing much of their previous influence and respectability. As a consequence a new religious style emerged, ". . .shaped by a desire to strike back at anything modern."[16] And in this union of social and theological reaction the foundation was laid for the formation of a state of mind that Hofstadter characterizes as the "100-percent mentality."

It was this "100-percent mentality," annealed to cutting hardness by the fires of doubt, that came eyeball to eyeball with modernism and rationalism in the 1920s. And the showdown was made even more dramatic by the end of the rural and small-town Protestant hegemony in America. The urban, industrial, pluralistic America had finally arrived.

There were countless minor skirmishes and several major battles marking this confrontation, and both the skirmishes and the battles frequently involved public education. The skirmishes were fought by groups such as the revitalized, Fundamentalist-oriented Ku Klux Klan, as well as by solitary individuals. And due to the already firmly entrenched tradition of local lay control of public education, many of them were fought in the schools, or elsewhere in the life space of some hapless teacher or administrator. How many of these skirmishes there actually were is impossible to determine. But the pressures of the times insure that they must have been plentiful. Unfortunately the incidents and participants now suffer the obscurity that history often reserves for those of humble status.

Compared to the skirmishes, the battles and the battlers are strikingly easy to identify and Hofstadter calls attention to three major conflicts: the rigid defense of prohibition, the campaign against Al Smith, and the Scopes "Monkey Trial"[17]—one of the most well-known incidents in the history of American education.

The only victory that the 100 percenters won was the defeat of Smith. And even this triumph was sucked of its joy by one of the results: the restructuring of the Democratic Party and its transformation into the political agent for the new America.[18]

Hofstadter argues that the wars were over by the time the Great Depression brought its profoundly disruptive economic conditions to America. But what the depression did for the vanquished was to rub their noses in the inability of their thought models to deal with this monumental turn of events. This final setback was too much for many of the losing side. Pushed out of their place as value setters for the entire culture and rudely treated after their displacement, many of them turned to fanatical opposition to the New Deal—and it was at this juncture that the direct forebear of the contemporary American Radical Right first saw the light of day. Squalling against the rudeness of the times and the rough treatment of the obstetrician, it hung awkwardly upside down in the glaring lights of modernism while anxiety over displaced prerogatives slapped life into its body. The 100-percent believer in the fundamentals, made passionate by the actuality of dispossession, had sired the 100-percent American.

Thus it becomes clear that Hofstadter has no need of the anxiety of the newly arrived, upwardly mobile individual of any social class. Instead he places his emphasis on the downward mobility of those displaced by rationalism. However, in this contention Hofstadter is not making a claim that is antithetical to those made by Lipset and Riesman–Glazer. But he does markedly redirect the status anxiety theme. Nevertheless he chooses some of the very same historical incidents and periods as being relevantly similar to the contemporary American Radical Right (for example, the fundamentalist-oriented Ku Klux Klan of the 1920s).

In view of the different thrusts of these various theoretical claims, especially when they concern the same historical event, it is tempting to assume that one of them must be mistaken. But such a conclusion need not necessarily follow. It is equally possible that they all are correct, but correct for only a portion of the individuals that are involved with the contemporary American Radical Right. After all, it is an extremely complex movement with many different, interrelating beliefs and groups. Consequently it seems likely that the individuals involved in these various beliefs and groups are the results of a number of different historical backgrounds and trends. Thus each attempt at developing the historical and theoretical facts about this movement could enjoy the limited success of accomplishing this for some of its aspects. Perhaps in the future, development of a general theory of status anxiety will furnish a badly needed synthesis of all of these permutations.

This brings us to the final and most important reasons for giving so much space to this one theoretical position. First, Hofstadter's interpretation of the contemporary American Radical Right emphasizes the interaction of the nation's history of fundamentalism with the modern pressure of rationalism. Such an interpretation places the Fundamental Protestant Radical Right, the subject of this book, in a central position. In this version of the status anxiety theory they represent a sort of missing link (pardon the Darwinian pun) between the old style sacerdotal fundamentalism of the 1920s and the contemporary secular fundamentalism of organizations like the John Birch Society.[19] Such a claim is much too relevant to miss. Second, even if Holfstadter is wrong about the degree of general significance of fundamentalism to the Radical Right, he still offers an excellent possibility for explaining salient features of its Fundradist component. Third, and lastly, it is in this particular body of theory that the historical implications are most clearly drawn out. As a consequence of this clarity they furnish an excellent opportunity to illustrate the relationship that such a theoretical position can have in choosing the relevantly similar from history.

There are entirely too many theories on the origins of the contemporary American Radical Right and its Fundradist component to tease out the historical implications of each of them. In fact, there are too many theories available to give each of them coverage. Nevertheless, each of these theoretical positions does have historical implications.

There is no totally satisfactory way out of this difficulty short of writing a book detailing all of the theories and another dealing with their historical implications. But since such an undertaking is not possible at this time, we are forced to compromise. It is for this reason that the status anxiety theory was chosen for detailed exposition.

Theories based on a personality structure

The Fascist and Nazi ascendance to power, the World War that followed, and the subsequent discovery of the atrocities committed under their aegis led theoreticians to speculate on how and why these movements had come about. Perhaps it was the particularly nightmarish quality of Nazi actions that caused some of the theorists to place less reliance than usual on traditional political, economic, or social interpretations. But whatever the cause, the result was a new direction in theorizing about right-wing extremism. This new direction featured the general hypothesis that right-wing ideologies were, in the final analysis, expressions of deep-seated, pathological personality characteristics. Later, the scope of this theoretical position was expanded to include extremists not on the right.

A theory based on the Fascistic personality type

The most well-known and time-tested personality theory dealing with the Radical Right is contained in the work of T. W. Adorno, Else Frenkel-Brunswik, D. J. Levinson, and R. N. Sanford, published in 1950 under the title *The Authoritarian Personality*. Growing out of a war-engendered analysis of the ideological content of anti-Semitism and a postwar analysis of ethnocentrism, this masssive study contained the first publication of the now famous F Scale (the F stands for Fascism) and the evidence underlying its formulation.

As in other personality-based theories of right-wing behavior, the major hypothesis of the Adorno position is that the "political, economic and social convictions of an individual form a broad and coherent pattern. . .[which] is an expression of deep-lying

trends in the personality."[20] More specifically, Adorno maintains
that authoritarian personality types display an abnormal amount
of respect for convention, are unusually submissive to authority
but arbitrary and harsh with underlings, admire ruthlessness, exhibit pervasive and rigid hostility toward stereotyped out-groups
and positive, submissive attitudes toward stereotyped in-groups,
profess political and economic conservatism that ranges into
pseudoconservatism,[21] are unusually negative and cynical, and are
preoccupied with nonspiritual matters.[22]

When it is considered that this study was published in 1950, before the emergence of the contemporary American Radical
Right, the degree to which the authors have succeeded in describing
personality characteristics that would logically lend themselves to
the formulation of the Fundradist ideology is truly remarkable.
Even the finding that authoritarian personality types are "preoccupied with nonspiritual matters" is not as contradictory as it first
appears. After all, one of the ways that a Fundradist can be identified is by his sacralization of that which is normally secular. The
most obvious conclusion concerning this tendency would be that
it is an index of the critical importance of the spiritual in their
lives. But if this sacralization were to turn out to be simply a convenient rationalization for dogmatism, it is not implausible to
conjecture that it is actually an ironically contorted index of the
nonspiritual basis of the movement.

Such speculation is given added credibility by another of the
Adorno team's findings. It seems that church membership positively
correlates with a high score on the Fascism scale. Moreover, there
was an even greater correlation between a high Fascism scale score
and regularity of church attendance.[23] Although the authors warn
against hasty conclusions concerning this finding it seems appropriate to reflect on it.

*A theory based on the nature of authoritarian
personalities, distinguishing structure from content*

The theory that guided the research reported in *The Authoritarian
Personality* focused on the Fascist type of authoritarianism. As a

consequence of this emphasis the historian using this body of theory as a point of reference would concentrate his research efforts on previous examples of rightist forms of authoritarianism. (An excellent example of this can be found in the work of Richard Hofstadter. In his essay "The Pseudo-Conservative Revolt" he draws heavily on the Adorno work and concentrates his historical research on the right.[24]) The difficulty with this is that there appears to be no shortage of individuals who seem to be authoritarian and intolerant but who are not Fascistic or psuedoconservative. For example, there is no shortage of such individuals on the far left. Indeed, the Adorno study has been criticized on precisely this point.[25]

But even if left authoritarians are included with right authoritarians there is still a fundamental problem. The dichotomy of left and right authoritarianism rules out the possibility that there might be other versions of the same phenomenon that occupy the political center or are outside the realm of politics althogether.

It is precisely this possibility that occupied the attention of Milton Rokeach. In his truly excellent work *The Open and Closed Mind,* Rokeach advances a deftly developed body of experimental evidence which indicates that authoritarian belief structures are *not* confined to the extremes of right or left. By making a sharp distinction between the content and the structure of the ideological systems, something the Adorno study failed to do, he has developed a theoretical position that is capable of dealing with individuals whose thought content is not extreme, but is structured in an authoritarian, intolerant, and dogmatic fashion.

By focusing on the general properties common to all forms of authoritarianism, rather than on properties unique to right or left authoritarianism, and by concentrating on the structure of individual human personalities exclusive of their political persuasions, Rokeach blazes new trails. And he presents real difficulties to the historian who would use his theory either as a guide or as a major consideration. Rokeach himself says, "Authoritarianism can be observed at any one time in history in a variety of human activities, and we should think that it would have similar properties whether it is exhibited by Caesar, Napoleon, Hitler, Stalin, Khrushchev,

Roosevelt, or Eisenhower."[26] He then suggests that what is needed is a deliberate turning away from concern with the one or two brands of authoritarianism that may be popular at any one time, and a greater emphasis upon a more theoretical *ahistorical* analysis of the properties all forms of authoritarianism have in common.[27] But it should not be assumed that such an ahistorical mode of theorizing cannot have major implications for the historian. It is just that their development would require an unusual perspective.

A neo-Freudian theory of the etiology of the
authoritarian personality type

By looking at authoritarian political behavior as a social manifestation of a personality type both Adorno and Rokeach tighten the focus of social analysis almost as closely as it will go. It is Else Frenkel-Brunswik, however—herself a contributor to the Adorno effort—who attaches the close-up lens and proposes a particular etiology for that personality type.

Her main contention, derived from psychoanalysis, is that early parent-child relationships lay the basic groundwork for the type of personality that finds authoritarian movements so attractive.[28] Specifically, these relationships are characterized by arbitrary and overwhelmingly authoritarian parents who demand total submission from the child. By virtue of his vulnerability the child is forced to adopt a pattern of compulsive conformity. In the process he is prevented from developing his own personal identity. He is too busy submitting to decide that he is anything that does not coincide with his parents' wishes. Consequently, self-reliance and independence are never permitted to develop.[29]

Frenkel-Brunswik observes that children who are ego-dominated in this manner frequently identify very closely with, and ostentatiously glorify, their parents. Nevertheless, the personal stifling that is required has the consequence of generating deep hostility toward the parents. Thus their common reaction to their parents is a profoundly disturbing feeling of ambivalence. In fact these feelings are so disturbing that they are not consciously tolerable. As a consequence they are dealt with through a reaction formation that stresses compulsive conformity and an intolerance for ambiguity, the latter being associated with the forbidden feelings of ambivalence.[30]

The parents' stress on self-negation not only prevents the child from developing his own independent self-concept, it also prevents him from developing a feeling of personal worth. He often feels worthless or depraved, but his insecure personal footing keeps him from squarely facing his own inadequacies. The result of this is that the individual comes to project his weaknesses and short-comings onto the social environment. His world comes to "contain" all of the problems, both real and imagined, that he is unable to deal with himself.[31]

Finally, because of the deep underlying resentment that this type of individual has for authority figures, we find him prone to easy exchange of his adopted political cause or leader.[32] Thus the "true believer" in a traditional religion becomes a more likely convert to movements such as Communism or Fascism than the non–"true believing" agnostic. (This also suggests a possible reason why Hitler continually looked for converts from the ranks of the Communist party during the early days of Nazism.)

A theory based on religious belief

Franklin H. Littel's notion of "social pathology" will be the last theoretical position examined in this chapter. It is a curious amalgam of Littel's religious convictions and facts derived from observation and comparison. It has been included for its novelty and for the fact that it places the Fundradists in a centrally significant role. It is *not* a personality-based theory and is not meant to be included in that group.

In his book, *Wild Tongues: A Handbook of Social Pathology,* Littel uses observation and comparison to derive a typology of "pathological" political movements. He uses the term "pathological" because the politics is of the totalitarian variety and he presumes this to be a sign of social sickness.

This typology takes the form of a fifteen-point "grid" that is to to be used as a tool for the identification of "pathological" movements. The fifteen points of the grid are given the following headings:

1. Anti-Semitism.
2. Ideological politics.
3. The politics of polarization.
4. Reconstruction of sacral society.
5. A new periodization of history.
6. A new anthropology.
7. The elite.
8. The cult of violence.
9. The inducement of social aphasia.
10. The police state.
11. Monolithic party and/or state.
12. The beautiful state.
13. The false consensus.
14. Reliance upon the oral tradition.
15. Determinism.[33]

Although space limitations preclude an explanation of each of these grid points, many of the titles are informative in and of themselves. Further, they do serve to acquaint the reader with the areas which Littel emphasizes. But the point critical to the inclusion of this "grid" is the kind of conclusions Littel reaches with its aid.

First, after placing both traditional Fascism and the contemporary Radical Right, including the Fundradists, on the "grid"; Littel concludes that the two are essentially the same. In fact, he suggests that the term "Radical Right" is a phrase used by writers who are reluctant to call it what it is—Fascism.[34]

Second, he maintains that a "grid"-based comparison of Fascism and Communism reveals similarities at fourteen of the fifteen points.[35] Thus, from Littel's theoretical vantage point there is more commonality than difference between the two *apparently* antithetical ideologies.[36]

Third, and finally, Littel concludes that both Communism and Fascism have a similar genesis. He says,

> Where such movements have come to strength or triumph, they have been "post-Christian": that is, they have gained

authority as the Christian movement has lost momentum and direction. Put bluntly, both Communist and Fascist-type movements are products of culture-religion in decline.[37]

It is at this point that Littel's own religious convictions become most directly involved. As a Protestant theologian he believes Christianity to be the legitimate carrier of the meaning of history. Consequently, what he believes to be a product of its decline, he regards as pathological.

Although such an interpretation is interesting, it suffers from being too narrow to comfortably accommodate those who do not believe as Littel does. However, his view does place the Fundradists in a position of great importance. In fact, just as in Hofstadter's theory, they provide the missing link. Being residents of the Radical Right (Littel would say Fascists) and claiming to be Christians, the Fundradists bridge Littel's gap between the legitimate sacral past and in illegitimate secular corruption of it. They represent the point in his theory where Christianity loses "momentum and direction" and becomes a "post-Christian pathology."

Summary

It is in the nature of a sampler that when the box is empty the appetite has only been whetted. So it must be with our review of the theorizing that is applicable to America's Radical Right and its Fundradist component. Inevitably, the question arises as to whether the selection has been sufficient for the purpose. Even within the rather limited selection available in this review there are positions that could have been profitably pursued. For example, the first point of Franklin Littel's "totalitarian grid" has to do with anti-Semitism. This contention could have been related to the theoretical position of Hannah Arendt. She maintains that anti-Semitism is endemic to all totalitarian systems because the Jew is representative of God, the true Author of history, that the totalitarian ideologues must deny.[38] Littel is in agreement with this analysis.[39]

At first glance it might appear that such a contention would exclude any ideology connected with Christianity; since this religion is obviously dependent on the position that the Jew was the bearer of history. However, anti-Semitism is hardly a stranger to Christian ranks. Furthermore, the Fundradist contention that America is the chosen country, at least of today, suggests that the theory might be more applicable than it first appears to be.

Thus, any stopping point is bound to fall short. For example, even if we limited ourselves to styles of thought, an obvious correlate of the personality dispositions developed earlier and only a position within a position, we would have to review the work done on ethnocentric thinking,[40] stereotyped thinking,[41] "narrow minded" thinking, and middle-class thinking[42] in order even to begin. Consequently, we are forced to draw the matter to a close with the reminder that the richness of these theoretical grounds is sufficient to give pause to the historian who would choose to lean very heavily on any one of them.

13

The historical context

Mindful of the introductory remarks that establish the connection between theory and history, what can be said about the way that the Fundradists fit into the historical context? Starkly and simply put, it is that in many ways their views are of the last century.

Even in its most general sense, being "of the last century" does *not* mean that the Fundradists simply have an affinity for it. Rather, it means that there are direct connections between Fundradist ideology and certain prominent beliefs and values of the last century. What's more, it means that these connections are unusually clear-cut. So clear-cut, in fact, that one cannot help but wonder how they have managed to survive the impact of modernity with their remarkable simplicity still intact. For example, they still believe that there is a simple explanation for man and his world, and that what men ought to do is abundantly clear. During the last century such a view was so common as to be the rule. Answers differed, but most were convinced that there *were* answers. Ordinary men had no doubt about it. And even such extraordinary men as Freud and Marx still clung tenaciously to the notion that rigorous thought could reveal the ultimate and elegantly simple

175

nature of reality.[1] It was the last century that would admit of such certainty.

The twentieth century saw simplicity and certainty die the death of a thousand compromises. For a while many refused to believe that these things had passed. But the evidence loomed so large that men could not escape it, and most accepted it in one way or another—although a few did not. The Fundradists are among those few. They still insist that they know the mind of the Maker.

The Fundradists' belief in "individualism" is specific evidence of the way in which they are reminiscent of the nineteenth century. They give this concept a restricted definition that involves laissez-faire economics, virtually unrestricted property rights, and the general noninterference of any *secular* government in the affairs of its citizens.[2] This echoes the socioeconomic beliefs of the simpler agricultural and commercial era that came to such an ugly end in the post–Civil War period that historians call the Gilded Age.

During this age the United States was transformed from an agricultural country to one of the world's leading industrial powers. For a time it was believed that this monumental change would be satisfactorily shaped by the prudent self-interest of the individual and the "invisible hand" that was presumed to give benevolent direction to a free market Adam Smith, an articulate developer of this economic view, summed up its essentials succinctly when he wrote,

> The natural effort of every individual. . .to better his own conditions, when suffered to exert itself with freedom and security, is so powerful a principle that it alone, and without any assistance, is not only capable of carrying the society to wealth and prosperity, but of surmounting a hundred impertinent obstructions with which the folly of human laws too often encumbers its operations.[3]

Smith was a Scotsman, and as such he would have found it extremely difficult to escape the shaping force of Calvinism, a theology whose influence on economics was without precedent. Before Calvin, Christianity had traditionally regarded the pursuit of personal gain as, at best, a necessary evil and, at worst, a sure road to Hell. Calvinism assaulted this view. It argued that the individual pursuit of wealth was not only permissible, but the duty of every believing Christian. Further, it taught that it was every man's spiritual *duty* to work. Sloth was viewed as a far greater danger to the soul than avarice could ever be. Finally, the possession of wealth became an index by which the Calvinist could measure the likelihood that an individual was one of God's elect.[4] This was so because the virtues of the elect were defined as diligence, thrift, sobriety and prudence—precisely the same virtues that were presumed to lead to wealth.[5]

This socioeconomic derivation of Calvinism was christened the "Protestant Ethic" by Max Weber and is part of the ideological soul of the Fundradist movement. Consequently, the fact that this particular ethic was tremendously popular and influential in nineteenth-century America counts as first-class evidence that the Fundradists' views are "unusually reminiscent of the last century."

The unusual popularity and influence of the Protestant ethic in nineteenth-century America was due to the convergence of several related factors. First, the United States was a predominantly Protestant country. Even toward the end of the century when the large influx of Catholic immigrants reached its height the country was controlled by an essentially Proestant power structure. Second, its emphasis on individual effort blended perfectly with the "rugged individualism" that had been spawned on the frontier. Third, its economic beliefs were afforded tremendous opportunity for realization by the relatively open society and America's enormous natural resources. Finally, the nineteenth century saw industrialization sweep the old agrarian economy to the background and raise a whole new structure of opportunity for the ambitious. All of these things were sufficient to bring faith in laissez-faire Calvinistic capitalism to the apogee of its power and influence during the Gilded Age.

Frugal, hardworking men like John D. Rockefeller and Andrew Carnegie rose from utter obscurity to become industrial giants. Railroads shot their track across the whole nation, and the mills that poured and rolled that track began to stick their smoky fingers into the sky at a staggering rate. Industries of all sorts sprang up, farm boys poured optimistically into the industrial cities, and Horatio Alger held up an optimistic mirror to Calvin's dour visage —getting reflections of young men who found their way to fame and fortune through hard work, sobriety, and frugality.

It was a time that would have brought the Fundradists cheering lustily to their feet had they only been there to witness it. For this was the time when the Calvinistic "Protestant ethic" that is so much a part of their belief structure had some basis in reality.[6]

Naive belief in the beneficence of the system was particularly strong in the decade that preceded the great railroad strike of 1877 and it continued to be the dominant point of view until the 1890s.[7] Not surprisingly, the Protestant churches gave massive and nearly universal support to this belief and, concomitantly, to the socioeconomic status quo.[8] As historian of religion Winthrup Hudson observes,

> Leaders of the churches may have disagreed on many things, but they displayed a remarkable unanimity in their approbation of the existing economic order and the "principles" or "laws" of political economy which provided its theoretical foundation.[9]

In supporting laissez-faire economics and the socioeconomic status quo these Protestant leaders were not *necessarily* giving evidence of reactionary tendencies or Calvinistic views. The period following the Civil War had produced unrivaled prosperity and the nation's wealth was increasing with each advancing year. Consequently, it was not unreasonable to support the status quo even if one favored the improvement of social conditions or if one were even relatively free from the influence of the Protestant ethic.

However, freedom from Calvinistic influences was not widespread among nineteenth-century American Protestant clergy. The Presbyterians and their theological cousins, the Baptists, were numerically plentiful and had direct ties to Calvinism. Even the numerous Methodists, descending from the ardent free-willer John Wesley, had taken on heavy Calvinistic overtones. Moreover, the "Protestant ethic" that had developed from Calvinism had soaked unseen through the tissue of most of nineteenth-century American Protestantism, leaving its influential residue in many places.

Perhaps the best way to illustrate the support that Gilded Age Protestantism gave to the socioeconomic status quo is through the example of two of the most famous ministers of this time: Henry Ward Beecher and Russell H. Conwell.

Henry Ward Beecher came from a famous American family whose members were so prominent during the nineteenth century that the human race was said to consist of "men, women and Beechers."[10] His father was the famous Presbyterian minister Lyman Beecher, whose sulphurous sermons reflected a relatively orthodox brand of Calvinism.[11] Henry revolted against his father's theological conservatism and, under considerable influence from the liberalizing influence of postmillennial evangelicalism, preached a liberal theology that gave great emphasis to God's love, the possibility of instant salvation through grace, and moralistic social reforms such as the temperance movement and, early in his career, abolition. In this connection, he also denied the hallowed Calvinistic beliefs in election, eternal punishment, and original sin and declared that the orthodox notion of God was "barbaric, heinous and hideous."[12]

But despite his very liberal theology, Beecher held forth with economic views that were anything but liberal, and in so doing he demonstrated the tenacious and widespread hold that the Protestant ethic had achieved in this time. Richard Hofstadter sums up these economic views: "He condemned the eight-hour day, insisted that poverty was a sign of sin, and urged that strikers be put down with violence if necessary."[13] To the pleasure of his wealthy Brooklyn congregation, he also sanctified the cult of business success.

Beecher's belief in the connection between poverty and sin is of particular interest. It is revealed in the following quote, ". . .no man in this land suffers from poverty unless it be more than his fault—unless it be his sin."[14]

This belief complemented the conviction that intemperance, coupled with a fundamental lack of thrift and prudence, was a chief causal agent in the condition of many workers. This is revealed in his comments concerning the large wage cuts inflicted on the railway workers in 1877.

It is said that a dollar a day is not enough for a man and five or six children. No, not if the man smokes and drinks beer. It is not enough if they are to live as he would be glad to have them live. . . . But is not a dollar a day enough to buy bread with? Water costs nothing; and a man who cannot live on bread is not fit to live.[15]

These sentiments stand out in curious juxtaposition to Beecher's liberal theology. Part of this can be explained by a commitment to Spencerian Social Darwinism that he adopted relatively late in his career.[16] But the fact remains that the primary importance of this peculiar contrast is its demonstration of the power of the Protestant ethic, even in liberal hands, and the extreme breadth of its influence in this age.

The Baptist minister Russell H. Conwell is our other example of Gilded Age Protestant support of the socioeconomic status quo and the pervasive influence of the Protestant Ethic. Combining the naive optimism of Horatio Alger with dynamic rhetoric, Conwell toured the nation, delivering again and again his inspirational sermon concerning how to get ahead. It was entitled "Acres of Diamonds" and is typified by the following admonition, "Get rich, young man, for money is power and power ought to be in the hands of the good people. . ."[17]

Conwell's famous speech must represent the ultimate fruition of the process, stated by Calvin, of turning the pursuit of personal gain from a soul-destroying activity into one that was a necessary expression of salvation. Note, for example, the following passage:

I say you have NO RIGHT TO BE POOR. . . . You and I know that there are some things more valuable than money; nevertheless, there is not one of these things that is not greatly enhanced by the use of money. . . . Love is the grandest thing on God's earth, but fortunate is the lover who has plenty of money.[18]

Like Beecher, and in keeping with the Protestant ethic, Conwell had little time or sympathy for the poverty striken.

The number of poor to be sympathized with is very small. . . . To sympathize with a man whom God hath punished for his sins, thus to help him when God would still continue a just punishment, is to do wrong, no doubt about it.[19]

Of course, the Protestant ethic is not yet dead. In general, however, its effect has been sufficiently absorbed into the nation's bloodstream that it is difficult to isolate it, or even demonstrate its full-bloom character. Moreover, contemporary happenings make its manifestation more and more anachronistic. This is perhaps best seen in the development of the "hip" counterculture in the 1960s and in organized religion's increasing commitment to social and political justice, ecumenical brotherhood, and the humanistic aspects of Christ's teachings.

That gets us, a little belatedly, back to the original contention of the historical segment of this chapter, that is, that the contemporary Fundradist movement is "unusually reminiscent of the last century." It turns out that their commitment to laissez-fair capitalism and virtually unrestricted property rights, as well as their militant opposition to all but moralistic social reforms, is deeply rooted in the Protestant ethic—a belief structure that exerted a powerful influence, religious and otherwise, in the Gilded Age.

This knowledge lends new significance to the fact that Carl McIntire, Billy James Hargis, and most of the lesser luminaries in the Fundradist firmament frequently sound like voices from another age. Now we know not only what age but what voice as well.

Sometimes the similarity between the pronouncements of men like Beecher or Conwell and those of contemporary Fundradist leaders is uncanny. Consider, for example, the following quote that appears in Carl McIntire's condemnation of the United Presbyterians, entitled *The Death of a Church.*

> The new confession [A reference to the Confession of 1967 of the United Presbyterian Church] nowhere recognizes that poverty is related to sin and the corruption of the human character. Solomon said, "He that tilleth the land shall have plenty of bread; but he that followeth after vain persons shall have poverty enough." (Prov. 28:19) All the social structures in the world cannot control the will and the disposition of a man who takes what meager earnings he has, or what gifts have been

placed in his hands, and goes out and, in one night, drinks himself drunk at the neighborhood bar, or proceeds on a Saturday
to a nearby race track and gambles it all away on horses.[20]

If the reference to a contemporary issue were not present this statement could easily be attributed to Beecher, Conwell, or any other
nineteenth-century preacher of similar persuasion. It's as if one
could close his eyes, listen to the Fundradists, and be transported
eighty or ninety years into the past, to the time when the "Acquisi-
tive Man" was taken to be a model of Christian virtue and the less
fortunate were presumed to be reaping the consequences of their
own evil and imprudent ways.

In order not to make too much of the influence of the Protestant
ethic, however, it should be noted that there is another important factor that is operative here. This factor concerns the relationship between the Fundradists' socioeconomic beliefs and their
conception of the ultimate cause of all human difficulties.

Edgar Bundy, of the Fundradist Church League of America,
was quoted in the ideological analysis as saying, "Sin is sin, in
any era, and sin is the root cause of EVERY trouble in the world
today as it was in 30 A.D."[21] This belief lends itself quite handsomely to support of the socioeconomic status quo, and to the
maintenance of the Protestant ethic; for if you believe that sin
is the root cause of *every* trouble in the world, it is not simply a
mistake but heresy to suggest that these troubles can be alleviated
in any way but sanctification. Obviously, you may succeed in
modifying peripheral conditions, but you will never get to the heart
of the matter in any other manner than through Christ. This view
is virtually universal in the Fundradist movement.

Naturally, once you believe that sin is at the bottom of it all,
the only kind of social reform that makes any sense is the moralistic one. And *how much* sense that makes is contingent on your
dgeree of hope for the future. This can be illustrated by again
turning to the nineteenth century for examples. In the process
another affinitive relationship is discovered between the Fundradists
and the last century. They are placed more exactly in their historical context and an important aspect of their ideology is examined
in greater detail.

One of the most important events in the religious history of this nation involves its transition from the aristocratically oriented Calvinistic notion of foreordination to the decidedly democratic belief that all men could be converted, charged with the Holy Spirit, and united together in common grace.[22] As with any other large-scale social movement, it is difficult to say precisely when this shift began or what, specifically, set it in motion. Suffice it to say that the nineteenth century was the time of its greatest prospering and that a whole host of political, social, and economic events were inextricably involved in its generation. However, there is one detail that is quite clear, and that is that the movement known as Evangelicalism was the principal vehicle for the expression of this fundamental change.

Broadly speaking, the term *evangelical* refers historically to that segment of Protestantism that emphasized the importance of spiritual conversion, the redemption of the world through the Gospel of Jesus Christ and the personal nature of salvation, while de-emphasizing the authority of the formal church and the importance of reason. Further, the term generally denoted those believers who relied very heavily on the emotional "revival" service rather than the formal, tradition-laden religious services that characterized earlier Protestant religious activities.[23]

Significantly, although Fundradists frequently vary as to denomination, degree of emphasis on any one item of belief, or other doctrinal factors, *all* aggressively assert that they are of the evangelical tradition. This, of course, relates to the fact that fundamentalism is intimately connected to evangelicalism. But, more importantly for the moment, it adds a new dimension of interest to what is to follow. For in the development of these historical details some interesting relationships are revealed that are quite crucial to understanding the contemporary Fundradist movement.

Nineteenth-century American evangelicalism had two ideologically distinguishable thrusts. The first, an optimistic form of Christian perfectionism, was operative from the beginning of the century until it metamorphosed into the Social Gospel movement of the 1890s. The second, an apocalyptic messenger of doom, initially trembled to life in the Millerite movement of the 1830s and 1840s, but did not reach significant proportions until after the Civil War.[24]

Traditionally, historians of religion have described the entire evangelical movement as an essentially conservative social force that focused the attention of men on heaven at the expense of social reform. Since the Fundradists are adamantly against any but spiritual attempts to reform society, it is easy to conclude that they are simply the last remnants of this socially reactionary theology. But the recent work of some historians of religion, which inspired the above classification, reveals such an interpretation as both wrong and significantly misleading.

Perhaps the best evidence that this is so can be found in the work of the religious historian Timothy L. Smith. He has developed a powerful new thesis which radically alters our understanding of these early evangelicals. It is Smith's carefully built contention that this movement was not essentially conservative at all. On the contrary, their optimism and zeal in promoting Christlike perfection in men and society, through individual salvation, played a necessary role in preparing the nation for a later direct attack on social ills. This direct attack began at the prompting of the Social Gospel of the 1890s, but it was the revivalistic evangelicals of the first part of the century that prepared the way.[25]

These early evangelicals' belief in the perfection of man and his society was rooted in a basic optimism about the possibility of actually bringing on the millennium before the Day of Judgement through mass conversion to the Christ of the Bible. Most of them also believed that this period of general righteousness and happiness would first be established in America—after all it was the greatest country on earth—and that it was just around the corner.[26]

Although the question of pre- or postmillennialism was not a heavily debated issue before the Civil War, if it had been, the vast majority of these early evangelicals would have been on the postmillennialist side. That is, they would have expressed the optimistic relief that the millennium would take place prior to the arrival of the Day of Judgement.[27]

Obviously this optimism about human perfectibility is drastically

out of step with Fundradists' beliefs. You simply cannot recon-
cile the kind of optimism that hopes to usher in the millennium
through converting the world in the next couple of years with the
kind of conspiratorial and apocalyptic world view that the Fundradists have. In fact, in many ways, the two world views are antithetical. Only in this agreement that America is some sort of
"promised land" do we find anything that suggests an intimate
relationship.

The optimism of the pre–Civil War evangelicals was so widespread that it almost drowned out the opposition. There was, however, one rather lonely exception who did achieve some prominence. This was William Miller, a New York Baptist farmer who
"got the calling" and began an evangelical tour of the country in
1833. Miller single-mindedly preached the same basic message
over and over again. It was that the millennium would not occur
until *after* the Day of Judgement and that this day was obviously
near at hand, for the evil of the world was increasing at a disastrous
rate. Somehow Miller even divined the year that Christ's judgement
would strike the earth; it was to be 1843.[28]

The evangelicals of the time pooh-poohed Miller's gloomy
prognostication. A typical reaction was voiced by Charles Finney,
the most well-known evangelist of the day. "I have examined Mr.
Miller's theory and am persuaded that what he expects after the
judgement will come before it."[29] It simply did not fit Finney's
characteristic optimism nor did it fit the extant evangelical persuasion. But Miller's cry did not, as most people expected, become drowned in jeers of derision when 1843 came and went
without the Day of Judgement's advent. Rather, it hung in the
air like a drifting bird of prey, waiting for its time.

The usual interpretation of the happenings in post–Civil War
evangelicalism has been that it switched from the postmillennial
optimism of men like Charles Finney to William Miller's pessimistic premillennialism.[30] However, recent detailed research on the
subject, especially the work of Timothy Smith, has revealed that
such a change was confined principally to the Baptists, Old School
Presbyterians, and a scattering of Methodists.[31] The remainder of
the evangelical movement still lay under the postmillennialist con-

viction that Protestantism's mission was to Christianize America in preparation for the second coming of Christ. To be sure, the carnage of the war had dampened the fires of optimism to some extent. But the evangelicals were still determined to build a great Christian commonwealth in America. Only now they had a new sense of the stubbornness of the problems that stood in their path.[32]

Slowly this new and more sophisticated sense of what it would take to Christianize America filtered through the fabric of evangelicalism. And slowly, as it did so, "the evangelical ideology of the millennium merged without a break into what came to be called the social gospel."[33]

Meanwhile, William Miller's premillennial pessimism was busily working its way into the ideological nap of those aforementioned Baptists, Old School Presbyterians, and a scattering of Methodists. Here evangelical revivalists stumping the land agitating for moralistic reform that would usher in the millennium were replaced by frock-coated harbingers of doom, who proclaimed that the nation was roaring blindly down the path to perdition and urged the few who could see "the truth" to repent before the judgement of the Lord was at hand. Here then were the apocalyptic premillennial evangelicals that once were thought to be typical of nearly all evangelicals of the Gilded Age. And here, also, are the Fundradists' ideological progenitors. To a remarkable extent they mirror the attitudes and beliefs of this particular segment of the evangelical movement.

But before we work out the conclusions that this narrowing process leads us to, it is appropriate at this point to develop the implications inherent in what has been learned while tightening the focus. The first thing that comes to mind is the fact that the evangelical movement in general harbored a belief that America had a special mission in the evangelization of the world. It will be recalled, for example, that the revivalistic evangelicalism of the early portion of the century widely endorsed the notion that the millennium would come first to this nation, and from here it would spread to the rest of the world.

This belief extended into the last third of the century. Even after the sobering experience of the Civil War the evangelical movement still subscribed to the notion that the nation had a divine commission. For example, in 1885 the evangelical minister Josiah Strong published a small book, *Our Country,* in which he claimed that America was the bearer of two great interrelated ideas —"civil liberty" and "spiritual Christianity"—and that it was the divinely ordained duty of the nation to put to use the "die" that God had made for the nation in order that we might "stamp the people of the earth" with our impress.[34]

Strong's book made a strong impression upon other evangelicals and it was particularly successful in sparking interest and enthusiasm at the numerous Bible conferences that were common to the evangelicals of that day.[35] Consequently, it is easily established that his view was a typical and popular one.

This fits beautifully with the Fundradists' conviction that the United States of America is some sort of earthly agency for God and that it is the final redoubt of virtue. Remember, for example, that Billy James Hargis describes the nation as ". . .one of the greatest gifts that God has ever given to man." And he maintains that, "What civilization there is now in the world is due to missionaries sent out from America."[36] These views, which are so typical of the Fundradist movement, are like echoes from this portion of the nation's past.

But what is particularly interesting is the fact that religiously nationalistic views were most popular with that segment of the evangelical movement that was the most optimistic about the possibility of perfecting society through spiritual conversion, the postmillennialists. The premillennialists, for obvious reasons, had much less use for it. This curious aspect of the historical context gets us to an insight concerning the nature of the Fundradist movement.

Very early in this study it was established that it is legitimate to label the Fundradists radicals because they advocate a massive reordering of American society (under the guise of returning to some sort of mythic Golden Age). This advocacy is heavily laced with vague promises about everything being put right when the nation regains its allegiance and obedience to God.

These pronouncements and promises are rendered quite peculiar by their juxtaposition with a formal commitment to premillennial pessimism, constant proclamations that this is the "end time," and stiff-upper-lip ministerial injunctions that, although the situation has obviously deteriorated beyond hope of recovery, the faithful must bravely continue to "occupy" until Christ brings the "Day of Judgement."

Considered apart from the historical context these contradictory pronouncements just seem to indicate the Fundradists' proclivity for muddy thought. However, when considered within the historical context, the contradiction points to the two greatest divisions of the nineteenth-century evangelical movement in America, and suggests that the Fundradists reflect both of them. Their advocacy of a massive reordering of society based on spiritual conversion and their religious nationalism can be seen to be direct expressions of the optimistic postmillennialist portion of this movement.[37] (This is not without a nice touch of irony, for this connects the Fundradists, through a common ancestor, to one of their greatest enemies —the social gospel movement.) Their gloomy prognostications of an apocalypse that will be brought on by God's people turning their back on Him are right in the mainstream of the premillennial pessimism that originated with the Millerites and was primarily promoted by the Baptists and Old School Presbyterians.

We see then that the Fundradist ideology is ultimately connected to the last century in a number of important ways. These connections find general expression in the Fundradists' commitment to the belief that there is a simple explanation for man and his world.

More specifically this connection is expressed in the Fundradists' commitment to individualism, which is defined in terms of laissez-faire capitalism and virtually unrestricted property rights—concepts that were the core of the socioeconomic attitudes of this nation during most of the last century. This ties in with the Fundradists' faith in the fact that anyone who really wants to can be upwardly mobile and their concomitant approval of such mobility and strong disapproval for anyone who challenges its possibility.[38]

The last century, particularly the Gilded Age, was the high-water mark for the influence of the Protestant ethic. During this time it came to be one of the dominant sources of values in American life. This ethic also plays a central role in the belief structure of the Fundradists. This demonstrates another connection between the Fundradists and the America of the last century.

Gilded Age Protestant ministers also "displayed a remarkable unanimity in their approbation of the existing economic order and the "principles" or "laws" of political economy which provided its theoretical foundation.[39] Fundradists advocate a return to this economic order and to their theoretical foundation. They also mirror the social attitudes that were prominent in the religious leaders of this past era—frequently, for much the same socioeconomic and moral reasons.

Nineteenth-century religious support of the socioeconomic status quo had some of its roots in the common conviction that *every* trouble in the world is ultimately traceable to sin. Such a belief led to the development of two related but differing religious views, both of which found expression in the vitally important religious movement known as evangelicalism. One involved a commitment to *moralistic* social reforms that were designed with the hope of bringing on the millennium right here in America. The other involved the pessimistic belief that the world was irreversibly evil and would only be altered by Christ's arrival to administer the Last Judgement. The Fundradists are tied into all of this by the fact that virtually all of them claim to be the modern representatives of the evangelical tradition. They also, paradoxically, exhibit both of the major views of nineteenth-century evangelicalism in the ideology, though they lean most heavily on the pessimistic premillennialist variety (which, not so incidentally, reached the peak of its influence during the Gilded Age).

All of this can then be nicely connected by the fact that the pessimistic premillennialist branch of evangelicalism, dominated principally by Presbyterians and Baptists, was the primary source for the beginning of the twentieth-century religious movement known as Fundamentalism.[40] (The beginnings of this movement were described in Chapter 2). Of course, this is precisely the movement that the Fundradists claim to represent. Thus the nineteenth-century historical context can be merged with more contemporary times.

There is much more that could be said about the Fundradists' place in the historical context of the nation. For example, their relationship to the theocratic state of the New England Puritans could be profitably discussed; as could their interaction with secular extremism in the present century. But space and time limitations urge a change of vein.

Before we close, however, there is an obvious yet vital point that should be made. The attitudes and beliefs described in the latter portion of this chapter were common in much of the last century. They also fit this world with a fair degree of accuracy. In our current age, however, they are quite uncommon, sometimes even bizarre. And they are often so inaccurate that their refutation involves reviewing the significant events of the last eight or nine decades. Put another way, possession of these beliefs in the nineteenth century was a mark of the middle; current possession is a mark of the fringe.

section 5

A concluding look

Having identified the major leaders and segments of the Fund-radist movement, dug out their historical roots, detailed their ideology, given a prime example of their actions, and reviewed a variety of explanations for the causes of same; little remains to be done. They stand revealed as grotesque byproducts of both Christianity and Americanism. Byproducts with an unhappy facility for successfully probing dark corners of the national psyche.

But just how facile they are in probing these corners is one question that has not been sufficiently explored. There is the possibility that the sex education hysteria was an isolated and atypical example of their ability to influence public policy.

One purpose of this "concluding look" is to demonstrate that this is not the case, by briefly sketching other examples of their influence. To be sure, the sex education issue is a particularly vivid example, but what follows will demonstrate that it was not and is not an atypical case.

The other function of this section is to provide a simple summary of the facts and to speculate briefly about the future.

14

Other influences on public policy

As was mentioned previously, the Fundradists' success with the issue of sex education was unprecedented only in degree. This chapter will briefly detail some other successes.

The items mentioned are not meant to be exhaustive. Such an effort would require prohibitive expenditures of time and space. They are meant, however, to be both representative and suggestive. That is, they are meant to convey something of the range of Fundradist influences. The preponderance of issues relating to education does, in the author's opinion, accurately reflect the Fundradists' concentration on this area of public policy.

Censorship

Radical Rightists have traditionally been involved in attempts to censor or ban books—particularly school texts. The Fundradists are no exception. As a matter of fact, they scored one statewide textbook censorship coup of unprecedented proportions.

In 1966 the Kentucky State Board of Education requested that the director of its Bureau of Instruction recommend suitable books for the teaching of Negro history. It took two years for the director's office to compile the list.[1] When the guideline finally appeared, it did not include *any* of the 200 books on the subject which had been recommended by the National Education Association. When asked about this omission the director stated that he feared "some of the books might be Communist inspired."[2]

This fear had its origin in a letter the director received from Dr. Gordon Drake of the Christian Crusade. This letter charged that 43 of the 200 books were "Communist-inspired."[3] Drake failed to identify most of the books he was referring to, much less document his charges. Nevertheless, the Kentucky director ultimately excluded *all* 200 of the NEA recommended books because of his "fear of controversy." There is no evidence that he ever checked on the substance of Drake's charges before adopting this solution.[4]

The NEA reacted by stating that Drake's charges were based on the background of the authors rather than any analysis of the contents of the books. (Drake had specifically objected to authors Herbert Aptheker and the late W. E. B. DuBois—both of whom had acknowledged Communist affiliations.) But then it began to back down.[5] Since the list had been *compiled* by a group of teachers from Washington, D.C., the NEA claimed that it was not their list even though they had published it. Then, in an even more unsightly curtsy to extremism, the NEA announced that after discussing a new revised edition with its compilers, it had been decided to delete Aptheker's books—not, they said, because they agreed with Drake but "to reduce criticism of the list."[6]

So, with just one letter, the Christian Crusade not only caused 200 books on Negro history to be eliminated from the recommended Kentucky Negro history study unit but got a bow of deference from the NEA. Among the "Reds" whose writings Drake later listed as tainted were Langston Hughes, one of the most outstanding black poets of our time and Gunnar Myrdal, author of the first really definitive book on America's racial troubles, *An American Dilemma*. One wonders what Drake thought fit to read.

Such massive success is not typical of Fundradist offensives for censorship. Episodic and almost incidental attacks are far more common. Typical of this approach is John A. Stormer's *The Death of a Nation.*[7] The book is an attempt to describe the decline of "Christian-America," but in the process it attacks several textbooks. For example, Stormer denounces Southworth's *History of America* because it describes the Normandy invasion as follows, "General Dwight Eisenhower of the United States Army came from the Italian front to command this mighty new United Nations force." (p. 769)[8]

Stormer alleged that this and similar captions on photographs lead young people to believe that ". . .the United Nations won World War II. They believe it because the history books have been rewritten to teach them so."[9] The fact that the allied forces were sometimes referred to as the "United Nations" during the course of the war seems to have eluded Mr. Stormer.

Stormer also attacks Magruder's *American Government* for allegedly encouraging the welfare state[10] and attempting to influence Americans to ". . .turn their weapons over to a super-government. . . ."[11] Stormer "documents" these charges with isolated quotes. He seems to assume that international government and a welfare state have nothing to recommend them and that textbooks should automatically condemn both. The possibility that a discussion of their strengths and weaknesses would be more suitable to American political ideals seems not to have occurred to him.

Precisely what effect charges like Stormer's has on textbook selection is very difficult to measure. Surely those who read and believe him have their confidence in our schools badly shaken. But it is doubtful that either textbook has suffered a significant boycott as a result of these attacks. Nevertheless, the effect of the sum total of all such attacks cannot be discounted. And the author's research indicates that there are many—most of them emanating from some segment of the Radical Right.

No analysis of Fundradist attempts at censorship should close without some mention of E. Merrill Root. Besides being an endorser of the John Birch Society, Dr. Root has written articles and made tapes for Edgar Bundy's Church League and joined Carl McIntire on the speakers' stand during the dedication of the

League's new headquarters.[12] His books are widely sold throughout the Radical Right and are readily available through several Fundradist sources.

Dr. Root's formal training was in poetry. However, in 1955 he published *Collectivism on the Campus* and in 1958 *Brainwashing in High Schools*.[13] Both books were meant as exposés of "Red" subversion in the schools.

In *Brainwashing* Professor Root largely confines himself to finger pointing at eleven American history texts which he claims, exalt "the common man," declare the U.S. to have indulged in "imperialistic" ventures, advocate a "world super state," and promulgate similar heresies.[14] He concludes that, "what American schools need is a thorough house cleaning."[15]

Nelson and Roberts, authors of *The Censors and the Schools,* conclude that Dr. Root has had "more influence than any other man in the attempts of pressure groups to rewrite American textbooks."[16]

The Fundradists and racial justice

It has previously been pointed out that an element of racism courses through the Fundradist movement. In the case of Hargis it is overt; in the case of many others it has been more covert; but racism, or a convenient rationalization of it, has been and still is there.[17]

For example, McIntire maintains that "racial brotherhood" is a false concept of Christianity designed by Communists to promote "class and racial strife in which the Communists delight."[18] He further believes that civil rights legislation ". . .championed in the name of freedom, actually restricted and denied to the people large areas of freedom that they had always enjoyed."[19]

This opposition to civil rights legislation, coupled with antipathy toward "legislation by the Judiciary" and any federal involvement with education has led the Fundradists to become vocal opponents of nearly every attempt to establish racial equity. In the late 1950s and early 1960s, this took the form of denouncing the Supreme Court's *Brown* v. *Board of Education* decision and all its ramifications.[20] More recently they have become active in supporting the antibusing movement and the establishment of "segregation academies."

Busing

Virtually every Fundradist organization in the country opposes busing to achieve racial balance. Such opposition follows from the nature of their ideology. But, so far at least, the issue shows no signs of becoming comparable to sex education as an opening wedge for the Fundradists to gain local recruits, money and power.

The most probable cause for this lack of potential is that opposition to busing has become a cause of the "establishment." This leaves no vacuum of public anxiety to be filled as there was with the sex education issue.

That is not to say that the Fundradist and their secular brethren have had any success with this issue. In February 1972 schools in Augusta, Georgia, were almost emptied because of a boycott to protest desegregation by busing. The boycott was reportedly organized by a group known as Save Our Schools, headed by a Fundradist, Rev. Stanley Andrews.[21] Andrews previously led an attack on sex education in Maryland and is closely associated with Willis Carto's far right Liberty Lobby.[22]

Liberty Lobby has been hitting the busing issue especially hard. It has formed a group called Action Now which is set up specifically to attack busing. Action Now leaders claim that over fifty groups have affiliated with them in this "anti" campaign.[23]

Segregation academies

In the late 1960s after years of delay and obstruction, it appeared that strict enforcement of federal court orders was finally eroding the last strongholds of racially segregated schooling in the South. But as this integration increased, so did the number of whites fleeing the public schools. White parents began forming their own private segregated schools. By the 1970–71 school year these "segregation academies" had become so common, especially in the Deep South, that "separate but equal" was in danger of being repeated under a different guise.[24]

Wide diversity exists among segregation academies in terms of their organization and support. Many have been established with the cooperation of local boards of education who have sold or leased public school buildings to them at very nominal fees.[25] In Alabama, Governor George Wallace made a great show of his fund-raising efforts on behalf of these schools.[26] But much of the leadership for actually creating the schools has come from the Fundradists.

Professor Allen D. Cleveland of Auburn University recently conducted detailed research into the origin and nature of these schools.[27] When the author asked Professor Cleveland if he had encountered many segregation academies that were associated, in some way or another, with churches having Fundradist predilections, he replied, "Yes, there were literally hundreds of them."[28] In fact, one thing that had intrigued Professor Cleveland was the large number of private schools called "Christian Academies."

However, Professor Cleveland acknowledged that his study had not centered on this type of sectarian school. Consequently, he suggested that his conclusions be checked against those of the research staff of the Southern Regional Council—publishers of *The South Today*. Robert Anderson, editor of *The South Today*, confirmed that his detailed research into the nature of segregation academies had convinced him that Fundradist type churches were definitely involved in a most significant way.[29]

These data should be tempered by the fact that many of these so-called Independent Bible Churches have no formal connections with any major Fundradist leaders or groups. There is, however, every likelihood that, with the exception of paticularly southern variations, their ideology is substantially the same.

In this connection, the author asked Dr. John Millheim, a former McIntire intimate and General Secretary of the American Council of Christian Chuches, if a significant number of churches either affiliated or sympathetic with Dr. McIntire were sponsoring segregation academies. Without hesitation, Dr. Millheim replied, "Yes, Yes, it is true."[30]

OTHER PRIVATE CONSERVATIVE SCHOOLS. In addition to their involvement with the creation of distinctly southern segregation academies, the Fundradists and other members of the Radical Right have started a significant number of private conservative schools throughout the remainder of the nation. McIntire's own "Reformation Schools" in Collingswood, New Jersey, are typical of this type of educational institution.

Westminster Academy, located in a Chicago suburb, is one of the most well-known schools of this type. It was started by Birchers and is operated by right-wing activist Dr. Phillip Crane and the Rev. Paul Lindstrom, a Fundradist minister. The John Birch Society also helped Rev. Henry Mitchell, a Negro Fundradist minister, set up a "Christian-Conservative" school in a black section of Chicago.[31]

While schools of this type are still scarce outside the South, it would be a mistake to simply shrug off their presence. The changing nature of public schooling, the deterioration of inner city schools, the various state efforts to aid private education, the possibility of urban busing to achieve racial balance, the increasing interest in voucher plants, and impending shifts in the methods of financing schools all suggest possible reasons for expecting these so-called conservative schools to proliferate.[32]

Prayer and Bible reading

When the United States Supreme Court ruled in 1963 that prescribed religious proceedings of any kind in public schools were unconstitutional, they also provided the Fundradists with one of their most durable auxiliary causes.[33] Thus far, McIntire, Hargis, and the others have not been able to manipulate and fuel this issue as they did sex education. But they have been angrily blaming the Court's ruling for an upsurge in crime, immorality, and general social disintegration while simultaneously pressing for various "prayer amendments."

The ban on prayer reading was greeted with widespread popular opposition. In fact, some observers believe that a majority of the public favored some sort of constitutional amendment which would nullify the decision.[34]

Many Americans share the Fundradists' anxiety over rising crime rates, civil disobedience, rebellious youths, and similar characteristics of the times. And they have already fixed some of the blame on permissive courts in general and the activist Warren Court in particular. Consequently, they tend to see the. prayer- and Bible-reading ban as a particularly outrageous example of the High Court's lack of wisdom. Unlike the Fundradists, however, they do not perceive the Court's actions as part of a Communist plot.[35]

Given these circumstances, hundreds of thousands have responded to campaigns designed to inundate Congress in a flood of protest mail. And some Congressmen have rushed to place their own particular piece of nullification legislation into the hopper.[36] From among scores of such proposed amendments, that introduced by Rep Frank J. Becker (R-N.Y.) emerged in 1964 as the leading contender. It stated:

> Nothing in this Constitution shall be deemed to prohibit the offering, reading from, or listening to prayers or Biblical Scriptures; if participation therein is on a voluntary basis, in any governmental or public school, institution or place.[37]

The first solicited deluge of letters supporting the Becker Amendment was organized by "Project America." This project, based in Collingswood, New Jersey, was sponsored by International Christian Youth, a subsidiary of Carl McIntire's International Council of Christian Churches. "Project America" produced over one million signatures on behalf of the Becker Amendment.[38]

The Fundradists intimated that a vote against the amendment was also a vote *against* God and *for* atheism. Since 1964 was a national election year, such a theme had broad impact. But its threat was diminished by the fact that nearly every major Protestant denomination, including the giant National Council of Churches (N.C.C.), was opposed to the amendment.[39]

Finally, House Judiciary Chairman Rep. Emanuel Celler (D-N.Y.), ironically utilizing prerogatives zealously preserved by conservatives, refused to discharge the amendment from committee. He said he did not think that it was possible to pass such an amendment without jeopardizing the Bill of Rights.[40]

Congressman Becker was unable to get enough signatures on a discharge petition and his constitutional amendment died in committee. The first effort at passing a prayer amendment had failed. Even with the support of millions of ordinary citizens and the adoption of a popular cause, the Fundradists had been unable to accomplish their objectives of overpowering the influence of the "modernist" opponents.[41]

In commenting on the N.C.C.'s role in this defeat, Major Edgar Bundy furnished still another glimpse of Fundradists' inability to accept the results of the democratic process or the good faith of those who oppose them. Bundy stated:

> . . .the National Council of Churches threw its weight in with the aetheists, agnostics, infidels, free-thinkers, leftists of all shades and the communists in opposing any such amendments.[42]

A measure of public dissatisfaction with the Court's "decisions in the area of religion and education is revealed by the fact that in 1966 nearly thirteen percent of the nation's public schools, and nearly fifty percent of the southern schools, were tacitly defying the prayer ban by continuing devotional activities. Additionally, some communities which had initially accepted the Court's decision began adopting resolutions that openly defied the ban.[43] This particular reaction peaked in 1968.

These acts of defiance often had broad-based support. But there can be little doubt that the Fundradists' and their secular brethren fueled the fires of this rebellion. The airwaves crackled with Fundradist accounts of the Supreme Court shoving the nation into the maw of "atheistic Communism." And these broadcasts pouring out of radios all over the country were supplemented by the sermons of local Fundradist ministers.

Thus, wittingly or unwittingly, the nation's self-appointed Jeremiahs of "Law and Order" helped create the atmosphere for open defiance of the law of the land. And in this context one cannot help but wonder how children can be taught to respect the law when their elders require them deliberately to defy it.[44]

Throughout the remainder of the 1960s there were various moves to revive the issue in Congress, principally the Dirkson Amendment of 1966, but nothing came of it. Meanwhile, the Fundradists had gradually downgraded the issue from its status as a major auxiliary cause to that of a perennial one.

Freedom of speech and the "Fairness Doctrine"

While the Fundradists have consistently been involved in attempts to erode freedom of speech, they have paradoxically taken the lead in attacking the FCC's "Fairness Doctrine" on the grounds that it threatened this self-same freedom. For years both Carl McIntire and Billy James Hargis have been giving the FCC a hiding for imposing a doctrine that they alleged could be used as a weapon to silence "real American" Gospel broadcasters like themselves.

It was previously pointed out that McIntire's WXUR was denied license renewal for, among other things, violating this doctrine. Since this denial McIntire has lost other stations that apparently feared a similar fate. While there can be little doubt that McIntire and WXUR did publicly abuse individuals without offering them an opportunity to respond, it is equally obvious that some of those who had him hailed into court were probably less interested in fairness than they were in silencing McIntire.

There is something odious about heaping verbal abuse on individuals and broadcasting it over hundreds of radio stations without ever notifying them or offering them a chance to respond. And there is a basic difference between the broadcasting industry and other medias in the sense that there is a limited supply of frequencies from which to broadcast. Nevertheless, recent attempts by White House staffers to "screw" their political enemies through misuse of federal agencies, clearly indicates that the "Fairness Doctrine" has the potential for becoming a major means of subverting the First Amendment.

Thus we are presented with the curious circumstance of having the Fundradists, who have demonstrated their contempt for free speech in a multitude of ways, serving to protect it by calling attention to a potential misuse of the "Fairness Doctrine."

The marches for victory in Vietnam

While there are many other examples of the Fundradists' influence on public policy which could be cited, there is a particularly vivid example which is sufficent to demonstrate that their impact can and does transcend the intimidation of educators and an occasional librarian. I am referring to Carl McIntire's public demonstations for total victory in Vietnam.

Since the inception of the war, the Fundradists had demanded that the United States junk its policy of limited objectives and go all out for a total military victory over North Vietnam. If this required an American invasion of the North or "bombing them back into the Stone Age" so be it. And if such a policy brought on the ultimate confrontation with the Soviet Union or the People's Republic of China, that was simply the chance we had to take.

This draconian position largely escaped national attention until 1969. By this time the war had become extremely unpopular with many Americans—so unpopular, in fact, that November of that year found some 250,000 Americans in the streets of Washington participating in a Moratorium against it.[45]

True to his career-long pattern of countering events he disagreed with an event of his own, McIntire announced that he was going to organize a Washington based "March for Victory" that would be held in April of 1970. He anticipated that "Christians and patriots throughout America" would convene "the largest demonstration in American history in behalf of victory over the Communists and for the preservation of a God-given heritage."[46]

Throughout the winter of 1969–70 McIntire mounted a lonely campaign to insure the success of his rally. He relentlessly used his broadcast network to promote support for the march, and slowly but surely this support built up.

Originally, McIntire had announced April 11th as the date of the rally. However, he had been informed by Washington officials that this date would conflict with the Cherry Blossom Festival. After initially bemoaning this "high-handed and brutal rejection," McIntire rescheduled the march for April 4th.[47]

Preparations for the march were proceeding well, when a most peculiar happening prompted a final flurry of confusion. McIntire discovered that a March 27th letter from the White House alleging that the march had been postponed had been mailed to individuals across the country who had previously written the President to protest his "no win policy." The letter, signed by Staff Assistant to the President, Noble M. Melencamp, alleged that an unidentified representative of McIntire's had initiated the postponement.[48]

McIntire angrily denied Melencamp's allegation, and suggested instead the White House was attempting to save itself political embarassment by sabotaging the march.[49]

At the time, McIntire's suspicions seemed likely to be a product of his omnipresent and all-explaining conspiracy theory. In retrospect, however, it does seem entirely possible that the same staffers who gave us Watergate and the other "White House horrors" might well have attempted precisely what McIntire alleged.

Despite the confusion, McIntire never flinched; and on April 4, 1970, the Washington Park Police estimated that 50,000 people marched through the nation's capital demanding "total victory" in Indochina.[50]

McIntire was rhapsodic over this, the largest public demonstration he had ever managed to organize. But if he was elated over its success, he was just as angry about the indignities he claimed to have suffered. These ranged from the alleged machinations of Washington officialdom, through the apparent indifference of the president, to the way the event was reported in the media. In fact, concerning this last category, McIntire was absolutely livid, claiming that at least 100,000 people had been at the march and many more had stayed home only because the media had engaged in a conspiracy of silence regarding the event. Then, as if to add insult to injury, the media had deliberately diminished the size of the crowd and refused him adequate coverage.[51]

Despite this alleged maltreatment, however, McIntire soon announced another "March for Victory." This one was scheduled for the fall of the year on October 3d.

During the intervening summer, comedian Bob Hope and evangelist Billy Graham cosponsored an "Honor America Day" on the Fourth of July. Although both men were friends of the president, they proported their rally to be nonpolitical. It was neither for victory nor withdrawal. Rather, it was billed as a day to reaffirm one's faith in the nation and to demonstrate national unity. It also served as a convenient opportunity for middle America to express support for Mr. Nixon's attempt to establish "peace with honor."

McIntire raged against Graham's involvement in such a compromise and drew invidious comparisons between the prior media coverage offered "Honor America Day" and his own rally. Nevertheless, on July 4, 1970, there were some 250,000 people gathered about the Washington Monument to support, in essence, something *less* than total victory.[52]

McIntire was undetered. He vowed that his October 3d rally would continue as planned and he pledged that upwards of a half a million Americans would participate with him in erasing the Graham-Hope inflicted stain on our national honor.[53]

Many thought that McIntire had given it his best shot in April. But on September 3, 1970, something of a bombshell hit the nation. Nguyen Cao Ky, the Vice-President of South Vietnam had agreed to be the feature speaker at McIntire's second rally.[54]

Headlines heralding Ky's acceptance blossomed throughout the nation, and Carl McIntire basked in the light of a publicity more intense than any he had ever experienced. But this glory was to last less than a month.

On the 26th of September, just a week prior to the march, Ky announced he had changed his mind and would be unable to attend.[55] McIntire hastened to Paris to try to rechange Ky's mind. But, he came home with the same negative response. Clearly an administration bent on winding down the war wanted no part of Ky's presence at such a rally and had managed to get this idea across to the flamboyant vice-president.

Despite the enormous pre-march publicity generated by Ky's acceptance, the second march was less impressive than the first.

Mrs. Ky who was to attend the rally in her husband's stead had her plane turned back to Paris by diplomatic and mechanical gremlins, and the Washington Park Police generously estimated the total crowd at 20,000. Clearly, America had lost its stomach for the conflict, and no amount of religio-patriotic posturing could turn the jungles of Indochina into the sands of Iwo Jima. The six hundred and fifty newsmen and television reporters from seven networks duly reported this fact to people all over the world.[56]

McIntire continued to try to mount another monumental "march for victory." But each attempt only bore witness to the futility of his cause. The crowds and enthusiasm dwindled as the war ground slowly to the conclusion of American involvement.

The precise impact of McIntire's "win the war" activities is very difficult to access. The results were probably mixed. His first several rallies called attention to the fact that Mr. Nixon's "peace with honor" was not synonomous with victory. This may well have prompted a prolongation of the war as the president tried an invasion of Cambodia and massive bombing of the North to gain better terms. But the whimpering end to the rallies seemed to indicate that even the radical right, for the most part, had had enough.

What is most significant is the fact that one man on the extreme right both religiously and politically had been able to get 50,000 people to Washington almost single handedly and to acutely embarrass official Washington with the promised presence of Mr. Ky.

Sometimes it takes a great deal more courage to be timid than brave. And if courageous timidity was what was really required in Vietnam, Carl McIntire did not make it any easier.

15

Summing up

The Fundradists are not about to take over America, either electorally or otherwise. But as the nation careens from crisis to crisis, its executive branch beseiged, its Constitution stressed, and its public sullen and cynical, their presence is hardly comforting. For should that "man on the white horse" materialize and arrive from stage right, the Fundradists can be relied upon to make every effort to bless and serve him.

A last word

It is difficult to avoid speculation regarding the intentions of the various Fundradist activists. Organizations built on "true belief" are easily exploited by unscrupulous manipulative men. In fact, should this be one's intent, then donning clerical garb and arming oneself with Bible and flag may be one of the most profitable and safe bunco games possible. Nevertheless, the subjective intentions of the various Fundradist activists are simply too intangible for responsible analysis within the scope of this study.

But while a conscious effort has been made to treat the Fundradists' intentions nonjudgmentally, there has been no need to extend the same courtesy to their methods. Time and again we have seen evidence:

> You don't realize what it does to you personally to have the innuendo that you are a Communist spread about. Now that is what he [Carl McIntire] did to us. . . . The point is the reaction to that. I can very easily see the reaction, the phone calls and the utter hell that people must have lived through when they, perhaps because of a liberal point of view on education which I may be opposed to, . . .were immediately stamped as a Communist or a sympathizer. Therefore, they had to endure that sort of reaction and even, perhaps the loss of a job.[1]

When asked if the phone calls included threats on his life, he replied:

> Oh yes! Oh yes! . . . I do believe that the mentality of some people, not all but some, that follow him [McIntire] can be highly dangerous. They would be doing a service in ridding the world of those who oppose him as a service to God, unfortunately.[2]

This ability to create an oppressive atmosphere of fright and suspicion has subtle but important impact on our nation. It imposes national and external restraints on public policy through fear of irrational attack. More subtly, it furnishes a nearly perfect excuse for inaction on the part of those who fundamentally favor the status quo.

In an open society, truths and values must be dealt with in a tentative, tolerant fashion. Values must be kept constantly subject to modification and improvement arising from each individual's sense of reason and contravening evidence. However badly our society does in this regard, we can ill afford to give attempts at successive approximation. The Fundradists demand permanently fixed values in a changing world. They want problems approached from an official position of ultimate truth while opposing points of view are ignored, suppressed, or treated as "straw men." In short, their concept of democracy is indistinguishable from totalitarianism. And this tells us a great deal about the nature of their movement.

It is inconceivable that a pluralistic society such as ours could give one religio-political view a privileged position, exempt from critical thinking without placing the entire society in grave danger of adopting a theocratic authoritarianism totally incompatable with freedom and individual dignity. Yet this kind of privileged position is precisely what the Fundradists demand.

Notes

Notes

Introduction

[1] Milton Mayer, *They Thought They Were Free* (Chicago: University of Chicago Press, 1955), p. 103.

[2] Ibid., pp. 166–67.

[3] Richard Hofstadter, *The Paranoid Style in American Politics* (New York: Random House, 1965), p. 73.

Section 1

[1] This is an actual example of Fundradist ideology which is explored in Chapters 3–6.

[2] Philadelphia *Bulletin,* Sunday, June 17, 1973, p. 1.

Chapter 1

[1] "Fundamentalists: Dr. McIntire's Magic Touch," *Time,* November 14, 1969, p. 81. In 1969 McIntire put his annual budget at the three-million-dollar mark. That same year Hargis totaled his budget at two million dollars. "Faith and Politics: The New Crusader," *Time,* August 29, 1969, p. 49. Since then McIntire has

suffered some reverses while Hargis has forged ahead. The author estimates that the total remains about the same.

[2]McIntire will not divulge the actual number of stations. In 1969 he boasted of having 600. A former intimate, the Rev. D. A. Waite, denounced this as untrue. Since then McIntire has acknowledged losing stations as a result of the FCC's denial of license renewal to WXUR, controlled by Dr. McIntire, for violation of the Fairness Doctrine. The Hargis broadcast data was obtained from Gerald S. Pope, editor of Christian Crusade Publications, on August 16, 1973.

[3]Most of this information was derived from an article in the *New York Times*, Monday, September 15, 1969, p. 51. It was updated and supplemented by the author.

[4]The evidence for all of these observations is available in the following chapters. It is not cited here in order to avoid redundancy.

[5]The lack of this gift did not hinder the Crusade's recruitment program. *Time* magazine, August 29, 1969, p. 48, indicated that the number of new contributors grew by 25,000 during this campaign.

[6]Wesley McCune of Group Research, Inc. (they specialize in studying right wing trends), states that sex education was the biggest thing for the radical right in 1969. Quoted by T. George Harris, Editorial, *Psychology Today*, February 1970, p. 24.

[7]Later chapters are devoted to the specifics of the sex education and sensitivity training conflict. The reader is invited to refer to it for specific examples that illustrate this claim.

[8]An extensive listing of various popular magazine articles on sex education and sensitivity training is available in the Bibliography.

[9]*Education Summary*, March 15, 1970. Quoted in the *Phi Delta Kappan*, LI:506, May 1970, p. 506.

[10]Specific evidence substantiating this contention is available in Chapters 4, 5, and 6. The quoted portion is taken from *What is the Difference Between Fundamentalism and the New Evangelicalism?* a tract published by the 20th Century Reformation Hour, Carl McIntire, Director.

[11]See Gordon Drake, *Blackboard Power: NEA Threat to America* (Tulsa, Okla.: The Christian Crusade, 1968), for a "gold" mine of such objectives. (Hereafter cited as *Blackboard Power*).

[12]Alex Inkeles, "The Totalitarian Mystique: Some Impressions of the Dynamics of Totalitarian Society," *Totalitarianism,* Carl Friedrich, ed. (New York: Grosset and Dunlap, 1954), pp. 106–7 (Hereafter cited as "The Totalitarian Mystique").

[13]According to the *New York Times,* March 26, 1968, p. 1, nearly 13 percent of the nation's public schools were continuing devotional readings as late as 1966.

[14]Ibid.

[15]Arnold Forster and Benjamin Epstein, *Danger on the Right* (New York: Random House, 1964), pp. xvi, xvii.

[16]Harry and Bonaro Overstreet, *The Strange Tactics of Extremism* (New York: Norton, 1964), p. 15.

[17]Raymond Wolfinger, ed., "American Radical Right: Politics and Ideology," *The American Right Wing: Readings in Political Behavior* (Glencoe, Ill.: The Free Press, 1964), p. 9 (Hereafter cited as "American Radical Right").

Chapter 2

[1]Joanne Zazzaro, "The War on Sex Education," *The American School Board Journal,* August 1969, p. 1, traces the beginning of the controversy to "a small group of California citizens" and then to Rep. John Rarick's (D-La.) congressional speech of June 26, 1968. The author's research indicates that Hargis' activities predate both of these events and actually set the stage for the controversy.

[2]See Chapter 7 on Hargis.

[3]See the *National Review,* October 25, 1964, for an article by Russel Kirk which describes Drake's firing sympathetically.

[4]This biographical material was obtained from a letter written by the Commission on Professional Rights and Responsibilities of the National Education Association, dated November 3, 1968. (Note that Drake, like so many others, entered the mainstream of the Fundradist movement by working for Carl McIntire.)

[5]Billy James Hargis, "Christian Crusade" broadcast, Saturday, March 2, 1968.

[6]Ibid.

[7]See Dr. Gordon V. Drake, *Blackboard Power,* pp. 94–97.

[8]Dr. Gordon Drake, "Christian Crusade" broadcast, Monday, March 4, 1968.

[9]Dr. Gordon Drake, "Christian Crusade" broadcast, Tuesday, March 5, 1968.

[10]Ibid.

[11]Ibid.

[12]Dr. Gordon Drake, "Christian Crusade" broadcast, Thursday, March 7, 1968. (It is of interest to note that in his Friday, March 8, 1968, broadcast Drake blamed campus violence on a "groundwork [that] had been laid with the aid of a fantastic network of controls" that permeated the education profession and was in the hands of a coalition of "lefty progressives.")

[13]Ibid.

[14]Dr. Gordon Drake, "Christian Crusade" broadcast, Monday, March 11, 1968. (This is paraphrased. Drake's actual words were, "Inside the classrooms of America. . .subversion is spoonfed to the innocent.")

[15]Dr. Gordon Drake, "Blackboard Power NEA—Threat to America," the *Weekly Crusader,* vol. 8, no. 19, March 22, 1968.

[16]Dr. Gordon Drake, *Blackboard Power,* pp. 131–42.

[17]In organizational terms, these early advocates included the National Education Association, the YWCA, and the American Purity Alliance.

[18]John Kobler, "Sex Invades the Schoolhouse," *Saturday Evening Post,* June 29, 1968, pp. 23–27.

[19]Cited in George Thayer, *The Farther Shores of Politics* (New York: Clarion, 1968), p. 147 (Hereafter cited as *Farther Shores*).

[20]Thayer, *Farther Shores,* pp. 63–68, and 159–63, describes the unusual history of this magazine and the enigmatic nature of Willis Carto. The *Mercury* became famous while under the editorship of that awesome critic of the "booboisie," H. L. Mencken. In the fifties the magazine took on a decidedly racist tinge when Russel Maguire bought it. This style continued unabated until 1966 when

indirect control was gained by Willis Carto, the secretive figure behind *Liberty Lobby*, a powerful secular Radical Rightist group, and previous activist in many ultra-right-wing activities including the Christian Crusade and the John Birch Society. Concerning the Liberty Lobby itself, Thayer, p. 160, observes, "The most notable characteristic of Liberty Lobby is its racist flavor." (This tendency is reflected in the pages of the *Mercury* in muted tones.) Beyond that, Liberty Lobby is distinguished by the fact that it openly acknowledges its political goals and pursues them in the lobbyist's traditional fashion. This puts the organization in the position of acting as an unofficial bridge between the "nonpolitical" entities of the Radical Right and official Washington.

²¹Capell's biography appears in *Homefront* (a monthly publication of the Institute for American Democracy, Washington, D.C.), vol. 5, no. 9, October 1971, pp. 64–65. This publication notes that in 1964 Capell was convicted of conspiring to criminally libel Sen. Thomas H. Huchel (R-Cal.). He was fined $500, placed on probation for three years, and forced to apologize.

²²Tustin is in the heart of California's Orange County, a county notorious for its concentration of right-wing extremists.

²³Frank A. Capell, the *Herald of Freedom*, June 14, 1968, as quoted in *The Congressional Record*, June 25, 1968, pp. 19027–29, by Rep. John R. Rarick of Louisiana.

²⁴Ibid., p. 19028

²⁵Ibid.

²⁶Ibid.

²⁷Ibid.

²⁸Ibid.

²⁹Frank A. Capell, *Homefront*, vol. 4, no. 7, July–August 1969, p. 58.

³⁰Dr. Gordon Drake, "Christian Crusade" broadcast, Monday, June 24, 1968.

³¹Ibid.

³²Ibid.

³³Ibid.

³⁴Ibid.

³⁵Ibid.

[36]Ibid.

[37]For prime examples of this basic thrust see Dr. Gordon Drake, *Blackboard Power,* pp. 131–42 and *Is the School House the Proper Place to Teach Raw Sex?* (Tulsa, Okla.: Christian Crusade Publications, 1968; Hereafter cited as *School House*).

[38]Rep. John R. Rarick, (D-La.), *The Congressional Record,* June 25, 1968, pp. 19027–28.

[39]*Group Research Report,* vol. 9, no. 16, October 21, 1970, p. 64. (For further details on Liberty Lobby see note 21 above)

[40]Ibid., vol. 9, no. 12, June 25, 1970, p. 45.

[41]*Homefront,* vol. 5, no. 5, May 1971, p. 41.

[42]*Group Research Report,* vol. 9, no. 10, May 15, 1970, p. 36. (This *Report* characterizes Rarick as "...probably the most right-wing member of the House.")

[43]Dr. Gordon Drake, "Christian Crusade" broadcast, Thursday, June 27, 1968.

[44]Dr. Gordon Drake, "Christian Crusade" broadcast, Tuesday, June 25, 1968.

[45]Ibid.

[46]Frank Capell, the *Herald of Freedom,* as quoted in *The Congressional Record,* June 25, 1968, p. 19027.

[47]Chapter 10 of this book is largely an elaboration of Drake's four-part broadcast—much of it being identically worded.

[48]Dr. Gordon Drake, *Blackboard Power,* p. 156. The Anaheim *Bulletin* is part of R. G. Hoiles' "Freedom Newspaper" chain. The editor is an ultrafundamentalist named Sam Campbell who acknowledges past membership in the Birch Society. The *Bulletin* played a central role in the nationally famous controversy involving Anaheim's "Family Life Education" program which ended with the scrapping of the voluntary program and the firing of Superintendent Paul Cook. For a well-documented account of these events and of the nature of the *Bulletin* see Mary Breasted, *Oh! Sex Education* (New York: Praeger, 1970).

[49]Telephone call to the reference desk of the Anaheim Public Library, Thursday, December 30, 1971.

[50]Dr. Gordon Drake, *School House.*

⁵¹Luther G. Baker, Jr., *The Rising Furor Over Sex Education* (Northfield, Ill.: Sex Information and Education Council of the United States, 1969), p. 2. (Hereafter cited as *Rising Furor*).

⁵²Dr. Gordon Drake, *School House,* pp. 6, 38.

⁵³Ibid., p. 6.

⁵⁴Luther G. Baker, Jr., *Rising Furor,* p. 10.

Chapter 3

¹Dr. Gordon Drake, *Blackboard Power,* pp. 13–14.

²Ibid., p. 11. On this page Drake describes these tactics as ". . .nothing less than blackmail on the American public."

³Ibid., pp. 24–25.

⁴Ibid., p. 130.

⁵Ibid., p. 142.

⁶Ibid.

⁷Ibid.

⁸Ibid.

⁹"Your Children Will Learn," Group W Television Special, April 3, 1970.

¹⁰Telephone interview with Mr. Albert Bobal, Principal, Westfield High School, Westfield, New Jersey, Wednesday, January 12, 1972.

¹¹Personal interview with Lorna Flynn, the Publications Officer of SIECUS, May 14, 1971.

¹²Luther G. Baker, *Rising Furor,* p. 1.

¹³Dr. Gordon Drake, *School House,* p. 2.

¹⁴"Playboy Interview: Dr. Mary Calderone," *Playboy,* April 1970 (Reprint).

¹⁵Drake, *School House,* p. 2. (Note that the second ellipsis mark used by Drake is incorrect.)

¹⁶"Sex Comes of Age," *Look,* vol. 30, March 8, 1966, pp. 20–23.

¹⁷"Playboy Interview: Dr. Mary Calderone," *Playboy,* April 1970. Dr. Calderone cited both of the above-mentioned tactics in this interview.

[18]Drake, *School House,* p. 13.

[19]For an excellent example see Mary Calderone, "Sex Education and the Roles of School and Church," *The Annals of the American Academy of Political and Social Science,* vol. 376, March 1968, pp. 53–60.

[20]Drake, *School House,* p. 18.

[21]Ibid.

[22]Ibid.

[23]Ibid.

[24]Ibid., pp. 37–38.

[25]This trend is evident in an examination of the number, type, and origin of articles on sex education in the appropriate volumes of the *Reader's Guide to Periodical Literature.*

[26]A 1965 Gallup Poll showed 70 percent of the public approving the idea of sex education in the public schools.

[27]*Time,* June 9, 1967, p. 36.

[28]Mary Breasted, *Oh! Sex Education,* p. 32.

[29]Ibid., p. 25.

[30]Joseph Bell, "Why the Revolt Against Sex Education?," *Good Housekeeping,* November 1969, p. 186 (Hereafter cited as "Why Revolt").

[31]Ibid.

[32]Note the chronological correlation with the beginning of Drake's anti–sex education broadcasts, Rarick's activities, and Capell's article.

[33]Mary Breasted, *Oh! Sex Education,* p. 36.

[34]Ibid. On page 80 of this work Miss Breasted describes the social and religious views of R. C. Hoiles, owner of the "Freedom Newspapers" chain and his Anaheim editor, Sam Campbell. When these views are compared to the Fundradist ideology outlined in Chapter 2 the resemblance is striking.

[35]Mary Breasted, *Oh! Sex Education,* p. 36.

[36]Ibid.

[37]Joseph Bell, "Why Revolt," p. 186

[38]Mary Breasted, *Oh! Sex Education,* p. 36.

[39]Ibid.

[40]Joseph Bell, "Why Revolt," p. 186.

[41]Mary Breasted, *Oh! Sex Education,* pp. 80–81, 127–28, 133–59.

[42]See "The New Sex Education," *Redbook,* September 1967, and "The Controversy Over Sex Education: What Our Children Stand to Lose," *Redbook,* September 1967, for an interesting example.

[43]Mary Breasted, *Oh! Sex Education,* pp. 124–25.

Chapter 4

[1]The author recognizes the breadth of this analogy. But a week-long comparison of newspaper clippings on *both controversies* in the libraries of the *Philadelphia Bulletin* and the *Philadelphia Inquirer,* plus other research along these same lines, strongly suggests that the dimensions, intensity, and, to some extent, the origins of both these controversies were similar. Of course, what the sex education controversy lacked was an equivalent of the Scopes trial —sharp focus. See Ray Ginger, *Six Days or Forever?* (Boston: Beacon Press, 1958), or L. Sprague deCamp, *The Great Monkey Trial* (Garden City, N. Y.: Doubleday, 1968) for descriptions of the Scopes trial.

[2]The letter writer is referring to Mary, the mother of Jesus, and the fact that Dr. Calderone does not deserve to bear it.

[3]Copies of these letters are in the author's files. The originals are in the "Crank" letter file at SIECUS.

[4]Details regarding the approximate time that Dr. Drake started this tour, the amount of time he spent on the road and the territory he covered were obtained in a telephone interview with Mrs. G. Drake reached in Minneapolis, the city of Drake's new "American College," on February 19, 1972. Other details were gathered from transcripts of some of his lectures and through the author's personal attendance at one such gathering.

[5]"Family, Schools and Morality Seminar," Arlington, Va., February 20–21, 1969 (a taped transcript).

[6]Ibid.

[7]David A. Noebel, *Communism Hypnotism and the Beatles* (Tulsa, Okla.: Christian Crusade, 1965) and David A. Noebel,

Rhythm, Riots and Revolution (Tulsa, Okla.: Christian Crusade, 1966). Observations regarding this second book were made in Chapter 2 above.

[8]Paul Putnam, Associate Secretary for Special Studies, Commission on Professional Rights and Responsibilities of NEA, personal interview, January 1971.

[9]The actual letters are in the files of the NEA's Commission on Professional Rights and Responsibilities in Washington, D.C. Paul Putnam, Ibid., can verify their authenticity. The author also has copies of these requests but has been asked to keep them confidential.

[10]George Thayer, *Farther Shores* p. 191.

[11]Mary Breasted, *Oh! Sex Education,* p. 10.

[12]Robert Welch, "The Movement to Restore Decency," *John Birch Society Bulletin,* January 1969, p. 23. The significant difference between the Birch Society's position on sex education and that of the Fundradists involved the latter's religionization of the issue.

[13]Ibid.

[14]While the notion of a "front" is commonly associated with Communist activities, Robert Welch has urged his followers to "organize fronts, big fronts, permanent fronts, all kinds of fronts." Robert Welch, *The Blue Book of the John Birch Society* (Belmont, Mass., 1958), p. 86.

[15]Robert Welch, *John Birch Society Bulletin,* February 1969, p. 13.

[16]Gary Allen, "Sex Education Problems," *American Opinion,* March 1969. (Gary Allen is a contributing editor of *American Opinion* and a former schoolteacher.)

[17]These mistakes and omissions are described on pages 82 and 85 of this chapter.

[18]Robert Welch had obviously given early consideration to the possibility of attracting non-Birchers to his movement through this auxiliary cause. In February 1969 he was speaking in terms of a 10 percent Birch, 90 percent "concerned citizen" figure for the Movement to Restore Decency. Robert Welch, "The Move-

ment to Restore Decency," *John Birch Society Bulletin,* February 1969, p. 14.

[19]*Homefront,* vol. 4, no. 2, February 1970, p. 16.

[20]*Homefront,* vol. 5, no. 7, July–August 1970. Smoot first attacked sex education and SIECUS in the March 17, 1969, issue of the *Dan Smoot Report,* then followed up with a five-week series of broadcasts during the next two months.

[21]Ibid. For example, the June 1969 issue of *Liberty Letter* informed the reader that copies of the "Rarick Reprint" and the long-playing album, *The Child Seducers,* were available from Liberty Lobby. The September 1969 issue of the *Letter,* headlined "SCHOOLHOUSE SMUT CAN BE STOPPED," told the reader "What You Can Do" to stop it. It also featured a front-page cartoon depicting a trio of salivating, barelegged men carrying valises full of "Filth," "Smut," and "Pornography," being pushed into the Public Schools by a leering man labeled "SIECUS and Federal Funds."

[22]Carl McIntire, "The Bible and Sex Education" (A statement presented to a New Jersey legislative hearing, August 14, 1969), *The Christian Beacon,* August 27, 1969, pp. 1, 8.

[23]*Homefront,* vol. 5, no. 7, July–August 1971, p. 51.

[24]McBirnie derived much of the material for this allegation from Countess Waldeck's article "Homosexual International," *Human Events,* September 29, 1960.

[25]William McBirnie, a transcript of his record "Sex Education," p. 12.

[26]Mary Breasted, *Oh! Sex Education,* p. 11. Although there are many fascinating examples of local literature, one put out by the Citizens Committee of California is of particular interest because it illustrates in an unusually bizarre fashion the dubious nature of much of this mass of material. When the CC of C's description of the Anaheim FLSE program is laid side by side with a position of William Shirer's *The Rise and Fall of the Third Reich,* which described a 1939 Nazi effort at sex education, there are a full six paragraphs that are virtually identical, with the exception of specific places and names.

²⁷Dr. Mary Calderone, "Attack on Education," *Vassar Alumnae Review,* vol. 55, October 1969, p. 5.

²⁸"Organizations and Individuals Opposing Sex Education," a list furnished by the National Education Association, 1970.

²⁹Ibid., and Dr. Gordon Drake, *School House* p. 37.

³⁰"Organizations and Individuals Opposing Sex Education" lists many different pastors and churches.

³¹The author has copies of this form from Mondovi, Wisconsin; Montgomery County, Maryland; Kalamazoo, Michigan; Racine, Wisconsin; Washington, Pennsylvania; and the State of Illinois.

Chapter 5

¹These data were derived from a compilation available in the files of the National Education Association's Commission on Professional Rights and Responsibilities, Washington, D.C.

²Ibid.

³Dr. Gordon Drake, a transcription of his "Sex Education" speech delivered in Room 2000 of the Jefferson Hotel in Arlington, Virginia, February 20, 1969.

⁴Files of the National Education Association's Commission on Professional Rights and Responsibilities.

⁵Joseph Bell, "Why Revolt," p. 184.

⁶Mary Calderone, "Playboy Interview," *Playboy,* April 1970, p. 2 (Reprint).

⁷*NEA News,* December 12, 1967, p. 2.

⁸Ibid., p. 4.

⁹Ibid.

¹⁰Ibid., pp. 7, 8.

¹¹Dr. Gordon V. Drake, "Sensitivity Training: Attack on Christian Values and American Culture" (Tulsa, Okla.: Christian Crusade, 1969), p. 40.

¹²He first made these charges in his June 1968 series of broadcasts, then in *Blackboard Power,* then in a pamphlet entitled "Sensitivity Training: Attack on the Christian Values and American Culture," and finally in speeches all over the nation.

¹³*NEA News,* December 12, 1967, p. 1.

¹⁴*Suggestions for Defense Against Extremist Attack: Sex Edu-*

cation in the Public Schools, The Commission on Professional Rights and Responsibilities (Washington, D.C.: National Education Association, 1970).

[15]One teacher told the author about a faculty meeting, held in the spring of 1969, at an elementary school in a very affluent suburb of Philadelphia. They were discussing where they might obtain family life materials for faculty use. A teacher suggested SIECUS. The principal refused to consider this possibility not on the grounds that the material was faulty, but that, if the source was known, it would likely cause trouble.

[16]Ernest Dunbar, "Sex in School: The Birds, the Bees and the Birchers," *Look,* vol. 33, no. 18, September 9, 1969, pp. 15–17. "Facing the Facts," *Life,* vol. 67, no. 12, September 19, 1969, pp. 34–39. Walter Goodman, "The Controversy Over Sex Education," *Redbook,* September 1969, pp. 78–94 and 193–97.

[17]*Look,* vol. 33, no. 18, September 9, 1969, p. 15.

[18]Ibid., p. 17.

[19]*Life,* vol. 67, no. 12, September 19, 1969, pp. 35, 38.

[20]*Redbook,* September 1969, p. 73.

[21]Ibid., p. 194.

[22]Ibid., p. 197.

[23]Carl Rowan and David Mazie, "Sex Education: Powder Keg in Our Schools," *Reader's Digest,* October 1969.

[24]Ibid., p. 76.

[25]Joseph Bell, "Why Revolt," p. 93, 182–93.

[26]The *Tulsa Tribune,* Tulsa, Oklahoma, Thursday, November 13, 1969.

[27]Ibid.

[28]Quoted in Breasted, *Oh! Sex Education,* p. 266.

[29]*The Philadelphia Sunday Bulletin,* January 18, 1970, p. 8.

[30]Files of the National Education Association's Commission on Professional Rights and Responsibilities.

[31]Lorna Flynn, Publications Officer, SIECUS, May 14, 1971.

[32]A fourteen-percent turnout in Anaheim despite national notoriety.

[33]The abrupt ending of this chapter highlights the precipitous decline of the Radical Right's ability to exploit public antipathy toward sex education. If the author's purpose had been an in-

depth examination of the sex education movement per se, much more would have had to have been said.

Chapter 6

[1]While this interpretation of McIntire's importance is based on independent research, it is a conclusion shared by many others. For a recent example see Erling Jorstad, *The Politics of Doomsday* (Nashville, Tenn.: Abingdon, 1970), pp. 27, 39, 57, 67.

[2]McIntire was awarded an honorary doctorate by Toronto Baptist Seminary in 1949 and has used the title ever since.

[3]Telephone interview with Dr. Paul Woolley, Professor of Church History at Westminster Theological Seminary and a friend and colleague of the late Dr. Machen, May 1971 (Hereafter cited as "Woolley interview").

[4]Clarence Laman, *God Calls a Man* (Collingswood, N.J.: Christian Beacon Press, 1959), pp. 18–20.

[5]Benjamin Epstein and Arnold Forster, "The Radical Right and Religion," (Anti-Defamation League of B'Nai B'Rith, Reprinted from the *1965 Christian Friends Bulletin*), p. 11.

[6]Laman, *God Calls a Man*, p. 27.

[7]See the January 22, 1970, issue of the *Christian Beacon* for an excellent example.

[8]Rose De Wolf, "The Sunday Puncher," *Greater Philadelphia Magazine*, August 1964 (Reprinted), p. 3.

[9]*The Philadelphia Bulletin*, Friday, October 2, 1970, p. 3.

[10]De Wolf, "The Sunday Puncher," p. 3.

[11]"Woolley interview".

[12]Ibid.

[13]Robert T. Coote, "Carl McIntire's Troubled Trail," A reprint from *Eternity* (1716 Spruce Street, Philadelphia, Pennsylvania), p. 3 (Hereafter cited as "Troubled Trail").

[14]Ibid.

[15]This circulation figure was obtained from the Christian Beacon Banquet program for 1971. However, Dr. John Millheim, a former intimate of McIntire, cautions that the paper is mailed to many whose subscriptions have not been renewed and thus

this figure cannot be used as an accurate measure of the size of McIntire's following. Personal interview with Dr. John Millheim, March 1971.

[16]For an example see the *Christian Beacon,* February 18, 1971, p. 3.

[17]Telephone interview with Mr. Daniel W. Smith, Manager, Christian Beacon Press, June 8, 1971.

[18]The minutes of the 3d General Assembly of the Presbyterian Church of America, June 1–4, 1937, p. 31.

[19]Telephone interview with Dr. A. Franklin Faucette, current Dean and Registrar of Faith Seminary and participant in the formation of the school, June 8, 1971.

[20]Ibid. It should be pointed out that Dr. Faucette is employed by the 20th Century Reformation and his estimate of the property's value may be influenced by this commitment.

[21]Millheim interview, March 1971.

[22]This material was obtained from a pamphlet, *Faith Theological Seminary: Training Leaders for the 20th Century Reformation Movement,* by Carl McIntire. (No date)

[23]Ibid.

[25]De Wolf, "The Sunday Puncher," p. 3.

[25]Dr. J. Oliver Buswell, a major figure in the ouster of McIntire, estimated that McIntire retained about a half-dozen churches after his loss of denominational control; telephone interview, December 6, 1971. Professor Woolley, a less directly involved, but keenly interested observer, estimated that McIntire retained the loyalty of about 20 percent of the denomination. This would amount to about 20 churches. Professor Paul Woolley, telephone interview, December 7, 1971.

[26]Ibid.

[27]Ibid.

[28]Coote, "Troubled Trail, p. 3.

[29]Ibid.

[30]Ibid.

[31]Ray Ginger, *Six Days or Forever?* (Boston: Beacon Press, 1958), p. 43.

[32]See Section 3 for details.

[33]See Alex Inkeles, "The Totalitarian Mystique: Some Impressions of the Dynamics of Totalitarian Society," *Totalitarianism* (New York: Grosset and Dunlay, 1954), Carl J. Friedrich, ed., p. 91, for an engrossing account of the relationship between belief in some "higher purpose" and totalitarianism.

[34]Erling Jorstad, *The Politics of Doomsday,* p. 35.

[35]Ibid. pp. 35–36.

[36]Quoted in Coote, "Troubled Trail," p. 3.

[37]Harry and Bonaro Overstreet, *The Strange Tactics of Extremism* (New York: Norton, 1964), p. 152. Note that "the chief function of the two councils—American and International—. . . seems to have been that of harassing the National and World Councils."

[38]Coote, "Troubled Trail," p. 4.

[39]Ibid.

[40]McIntire repeatedly denies that he is "political." But it is demonstrated in Chapter 10 that his movement attempts to sacralize *every* aspect of human existence *and* to radically alter American politics to fit this change. Perhaps his denial has more to do with the nature of the Income Tax Laws than anything else.

[41]The intermingling of Fundamentalism and religious nationalism is treated in a number of sources. See Erling Jorstad, *The Politics of Doomsday,* pp. 24–26, for one that relates this intermingling to the modern-day Fundradists. See John P. Roche, *The Quest for the Dream* (New York: Macmillan, 1963), pp. 50–75, for an excellent summary of the "Great Red Scare."

[42]Winrod founded the "Defenders of the Christian Faith," Pelley fathered the Fascistic "Silver Shirts" and Smith's activities ranged from the "Silver Shirts" through Huey Long to Father Coughlin and beyond. See also Donald Strong, *Organized Anti-Semitism in America* (Washington, D.C.: American Council on Public Affairs, 1941), John P. Roche, *The Quest For the Dream,* pp. 103–83 and George Thayer, *Farther Shores.*

[43]John P. Roche, *The Quest for the Dream,* pp. 158–83, provides an excellent account of the failure of this movement. See p. 77 for details on the manner in which the "Yahoos" association with Nazism precipitated their fall.

[44]These terms are Richard Hofstadter's, *The Paranoid Style in American Politics,* p. 131.

[45]Carl McIntire, *Author of Liberty* (Collingswood, New Jersey: Christian Beacon Press, 1946).

[46]Chapter 2, above. See also Erling Jorstad, *The Politics of Doomsday,* pp. 46–51.

[47]Alex Inkeles, "The Totalitarian Mystique," p. 91, maintains that "*the* characteristic of the totalitarian is that he sees the state as an institution with no right to existence in itself, but rather as a mere tool serving the attainment of some higher goal which is above the state." (Emphasis added.)

[48]Erling Jorstad, *The Politics of Doomsday,* pp. 50–55.

[49]The tract, "How Red is the National Council of Churches?" published by McIntire in collaboration with Verne Kaub and researched by J. B. Matthews of McCarthy fame, is typical of the tack that McIntire began to follow during this period.

[50]Jorstad, *The Politics of Doomsday,* pp. 53–54, details this cooperation.

[51]Charles Silberman, *Crisis in the Classroom* (New York: Random House, 1970), pp. 39–40, notes that the press frequently confuses objectivity with the avoidance of making any judgments. Consequently, they frequently report charges of such things as treason or subversion without comment, even though they know them to be false or grossly exaggerated. He also remarks that Sen. Joseph R. McCarthy understood this tendency and used it well.

[52]This biographical material was obtained from Bundy, Edgar C., Major, USAF Reserve, Wheaton, Illinois, Group Research, Incorporated, February 11, 1963, p. 1.

[53]Jorstad, *The Politics of Doomsday,* pp. 73–74; *Christian Beacon,* May 19, 1949.

[54]Thayer, *Farther Shores,* p. 260; Forster and Epstein, *Danger on the Right,* p. 146.

[55]Forster and Epstein, *Danger on the Right,* p. 147. Bundy made his attack on the Girl Scouts through the Illinois American Legion—an organization in which he had considerable influence.

[56]Jorstad, *The Politics of Doomsday,* p. 74.

[57]Ibid.

58Thayer, *Farther Shores,* p. 218.

59Jorstad, *The Politics of Doomsday,* p. 70.

60Billy James Hargis, radio broadcast, WXUR, Media, Pennsylvania, July 16, 1971.

61Quoted in Jorstad, *The Politics of Doomsday,* p. 52.

62Thayer, *Farther Shores,* p. 220; Forster and Epstein, *Danger on the Right,* p. 78.

63Thayer, *Farther Shores,* p. 218.

64Jorstad, *The Politics of Doomsday,* p. 71.

65Quoted in Overstreet and Overstreet, *The Strange Tactics of Extremism,* p. 190.

66Jorstad, *The Politics of Doomsday,* p. 71.

67It should be noted that the 1930s saw a great deal of right-wing activity on the radio. Father Coughlin was probably the best-known example.

68This biographical sketch is a compilation of material available in Thayer, *Farther Shores,* pp. 246–48 and Forster and Epstein, *Danger on the Right,* pp. 49–54.

69Thayer, *Farther Shores,* p. 247.

70Forster and Epstein, *Danger on the Right,* p. 50.

71Thayer, *Farther Shores,* p. 247, cites the year of his return as 1953, but Forster and Epstein, *Danger on the Right,* p. 51, reporting it as 1952, back it up with greater detail.

72Quoted in Forster and Epstein, *Danger on the Right,* p. 51.

73Quoted in Ibid. and Thayer, *Farther Shores,* p. 248.

74Overstreet, *The Strange Tactics of Extremism,* pp. 53–62, provides an excellent account of the nature of these "schools."

75Although available evidence indicates that the increasingly political nature of McIntire's ideology was a significant factor in denominational and individual defections from his movement, it is difficult to isolate the impact of this one factor. This difficulty is compounded by the fact that the direction of McIntire's politicalization complemented his autocratic style of leadership. Still, in all, there was a discernible trend in the growth of dissatisfaction with McIntire. In the beginning the chief complaint centered on his style of leadership. But as the years passed, the discontent became more and more involved with the political direction that the movement was taking.

These conclusions are based on the author's independent research and telephone interviews with Dr. J. Oliver Bushwell, December 6, 1971, and Professor Paul Woolley, December 7, 1971. Both of these gentlemen were intimately acquainted with the events described and agree that this was the pattern that the discontent tended to follow.

[76]Coote, "Troubled Trail," p. 4.

[77]Overstreet, *The Strange Tactics of Extremism,* p. 190. White is quoted in Overstreet as saying, "We set up Hargis along the same pattern as Roberts. . ."

[78]His general method was, and still is, to maintain that Communism has instigated an "artificial" problem regarding segregation and racism, in order to divide and conquer America. There is an excellent summary of this trend in Overstreet, *The Strange Tactics of Extremism,* pp. 196–98.

[79]Group Research, Inc., Special Report #16, Sept. 1, 1964, "The Finances of the Right Wing: A Study of the Size and Sources of Income of 30 Selected Operations," p. 7 (Hereafter cited as "Finances-Right Wing").

[80]Jorstad, *The Politics of Doomsday,* pp. 87–88.

[81]Ibid., p. 68.

[82]Group Research, Inc., "Finances-Right Wing," pp. 7–8. Since McIntire will not divulge his organization's financial affairs, Group Research estimated these figures using a rather sophisticated technique. See p. 19 of the report for computational details.

[83]Forster and Epstein, *Danger on the Right,* p. 101, cite the number of stations in 1964 as 577. Although this figure agrees with McIntire's last available program log, it may have been inflated. The *Philadelphia Inquirer,* February 14, 1971, p. 2, quotes Dr. D. A. Waite, an "associate" of the broadcast from 1965–68, as saying that McIntire's claim of 600 stations is "the greatest, biggest lie McIntire's permitted to go forth from his organization for so many years." Along this same line, the money for financing these programs comes largely from small individual contributions

and local committees of contributors. In the above cited article, Waite charges that "When people from one station collect funds and send them to Collingswood for their local station, many times the funds are diverted in Collingswood and the local program goes off the air. . . . How can he with a straight face talk about righteousness?"

[84]Thayer, *Farther Shores,* p. 243.

[85]The *New York Times,* Monday, September 15, 1969, p. 51, quotes McIntire as saying, "Radio is the mainstay of the whole operation."

[86]Group Research, Inc., "Finances-Right Wing," p. 4, reveals this surge in its computation of the total yearly earnings of 30 selected Radical Rightist organizations for 1955–63. (Note unusual growth in 1960–61, coinciding with Kennedy's election.) 1955—$3.0 million; 1956—$3.4 million (15 percent); 1957—$4.1 million (22 percent); 1958—$4.9 million (15 percent); 1959—$5.8 million (18 percent); 1960—$7.6 million (31 percent); 1961—$10.8 million (42 percent); 1962—$12.2 million (13 percent); 1963—$14.3 million (17 percent).

[87]Daniel Bell, *The Radical Right* (New York: Doubleday, 1963), Daniel Bell, ed., p. x., describes McCarthy as an "Unstürnmensch"—literally a "wrecker."

[88]This is not the place to work out the many and complex reasons for this right-wing surge. The speculation available in various disciplines is rich and varied and each contain its element of relevance. Of course, the content of the ideology (see Section 3) suggests much, as do the theories outlined in Chapter 13 even more.

[89]Jorstad, *The Politics of Doomsday,* p. 67.

[90]Ibid., p. 122, quotes the June 23, 1966, *Christian Beacon,* p. 3, as saying "Since 1960 sweeping changes in the growth and outreach of the Twentieth Century Reformation Movement, paralleling in many ways the changes and development of the worldwide political conservative movement have unfolded."

[91]Ibid., pp. 102–55. The author is deeply indebted to Prof. Jorstad's analysis of this union.

[92]Forster and Epstein, *Danger on the Right,* p. 105.

[93]Ibid.

[94]The *Christian Beacon,* September 28, 1967, p. 1.

[95]*Life,* July 16, 1972, p. 50.

[96]The price was obtained from the Cape May City Tax Assessor's records, August 4, 1971.

[97]The *Christian Beacon,* Thursday, January 21, 1971, pp. 1, 8. It should be noted that McIntire raised the money for beginning this complex *after* Shelton's accreditation problems had grown to monumental proportions. In fact, the College's jeopardy was the basis of the appeal. Now he points to the idle buildings as examples of "liberal intolerance and persecution."

[98]Decision by the United States Court of Appeals for the District of Columbia Circuit, September 25, 1972, p. 61.

[99]Ibid., pp. 70–71.

[100]The *Philadelphia Bulletin,* September 3, 1973, p. 1.

[101]The *Philadelphia Inquirer,* September 3, 1973, p. 1.

[102]See the July and August 1973 issues of the *Christian Beacon* for this evidence.

[103]"McIntire Attempts ACCC Seizure," The *Baptist Bulletin,* December 1970, p. 6.

[104]Millheim interview This account is confirmed by the *Baptist Bulletin,* December 1970, and by *Christianity Today,* December 4, 1970, p. 235.

[105]*Accent! ! !,* October 1970, p. 3., an editorial by Dr. John F. Millheim.

[106]McIntire goes to great lengths to explain that only the northern portion of Cape Canaveral was renamed Cape Kenndey and that his designation of his portion of the Cape is correct. (Since then, the entire Cape has been renamed "Canaveral.")

[107]The *Philadelphia Inquirer,* September 3, 1973, p. 2.

[108]Ibid.

[109]The *Christian Beacon,* Thursday, December 31, 1970, p. 5.

[110]Ibid.

[111]Carl McIntire, radio broadcast, WXUR, Media, Pennsylvania, January 27, 1970.

[112]The *Philadelphia Inquirer,* September 3, 1973, p. 2.

[113]Group Research Inc., "Finances-Right Wing," p. 7.

Chapter 7

[1]The term "analytic" is *not* being used in its technical, philosophical meaning. Rather, it is meant to convey the notion of getting at the foundations, essence or nature of a thing.

[2]Group Research Inc., Special Report #11, "Dr. Billy James Hargis, his Christian Crusade, his Christian Echoes National Ministry, and Connections with other groups," November 10, 1962 (Hereafter cited as "Hargis"), p. 4; and Forster and Epstein, *Danger on the Right,* p. 110.

[3]Group Research Inc., "Finances-Right Wing," p. 7.

[4]One produced in October 1962 called the National Education Association "a left-wing radical group." This was the beginning of a campaign against the NEA that has continued intermittently to date. Quoted in Group Research Inc., "Hargis," p. 9.

[5]Ibid., pp. 4–9.

[6]"What? Why? Who? Where? and How is Christian Crusade?" (Tulsa, Okla.: *Christian Crusade,* no date), a tract.

[7]Group Research Inc., "Hargis," pp. 11–12, 15.

[8]"The Radical Right and Religion," The *Christian Friends Bulletin* (Published by the Anti-Defamation League of B'nai B'rith), September 1965, vol. 22, no. 3, p. 10.

[9]Kennedy's candidacy and election may have created unusually high "Crusade" incomes in 1960 and 1961, thus led to overextension. Hargis attributed the decline in income to hostile articles in the liberal press. He also spoke of how he turned to Gen. Edwin Walker in desperation and how they landed a whirlwind series of meetings, "operation Midnight Ride," to help them get back in the black. Thayer, *Farther Shores,* p. 234; Forster and Epstein, *Danger on the Right* pp. 84–85.

[10]Actually it not only recovered but rose considerably above the bumper year 1961.

[11]Group Research Inc., "Finances-Right Wing," p. 28.

[12]Ibid.

[13]John Redekop, *The American Far Right,* Grand Rapids, Michigan: Eerdmans, 1968. 331 pp. 92–93. See also Chapter 10, above, for an analysis of this claim and of how it lends itself to the expression of covert racism.

[14]De Wolf, "The Sunday Puncher," p. 5.

[15]The *New York Times,* November 17, 1964, p. 2.

[16]Hargis relates the revocation to his support of the Becker Amendment in a letter to his followers dated June 11, 1965. The government's charges were considerably broader. But, nevertheless, it was clearly true that the Crusade's support of the Becker Amendment *was* a central issue. See Thayer, *Farther Shores,* p. 235.

[17]Billy James Hargis, radio broadcast, WXUR, Media, Pennsylvania, August 9, 1971.

[18]Thayer, *Farther Shores,* p. 236.

[19]Ibid., p. 222.

[20]Ibid., pp. 223–24. Not all of these "educational" activities require tuition. For example, the "Preachers' Seminar," usually held in May of each year, provides lodging and instruction in addition to a free library. Hargis appeals to his followers to fund this activity.

[21]The *New York Times,* August 6, 1971, p. 2.

[22]Forster and Epstein, *Danger on the Right,* p. 86.

[23]"Gospel According to Billy," *Newsweek,* August 24, 1964, p. 21.

[24]Quote in records of Group Research Inc., 1404 New York Avenue, N.W., Washington, D.C.

[25]Thayer, *Farther Shores,* p. 221.

[26]"Faith and Politics: The New Crusader," *Time* August 29, 1969, p. 49.

[27]Telephone Interview, Mr. Gerald Pope, August 16, 1970.

[28]Ibid.

[29]*Time,* August 29, 1969, p. 49.

[30]Peter Schrag, "America's Other Radicals," *Harpers,* August 1970, p. 37.

[31]Group Research Report, March 9, 1970, Vol. 9, #5, p. 20.

[32]Pope interview.

Chapter 8

[1]Quoted in "The Radical Right and Religion," The *Christian Friends Bulletin,* p. 5.

[2]Group Research Inc., "Finances-Right Wing," p. 7.

[3]Thayer, *Farther Shores,* p. 248; also U.S. House of Representatives Committee on Un-American Activities, *International Communism* (Staff Consultation with Frederick Charles Schwarz), 85th Congress, 1st session, May 29, 1957, p. 14.

[4]Group Research Inc., "Finances-Right Wing," p. 7.

[5]Dr. Fred Schwarz, *You Can Trust the Communists (To Be Communists),* (Englewood Cliffs, N. J.: Prentice-Hall, 1960). The book has sold over a million copies.

[6]Group Research Inc., "Finances-Right Wing," p. 5.

[7]Income figures from the Internal Revenue Service, "Exempt Organizations File," Form 990–A, "Christian Anti-Communist Crusade."

[8]Thayer, *Farther Shores,* p. 246.

[9]John Redekop. *The American Far Right,* Grand Rapids, Mich.: Eerdmans, 1968, p. 69.

[10]Jordstad, *The Politics of Doomsday,* pp. 69–70; summarized from his article, "The Remodeled Right: Schwarz and Stormer on Campus," *Motive,* vol. 26, November 1965, pp. 29–32.

[11]Thayer, *Farther Shores,* p. 247.

[12]Group Research Report, vol. 9, no. 14, July 31, 1970, p. 55; and Group Research Report, vol. 9, no. 2, January 20, 1970.

[13]Raymond E. Wolfinger, et al., "America's Radical Right: Politics and Ideology," *The American Right Wing: Readings in Political Behavior,* Robert Schoenberger, ed. (New York: Holt, Rinehart and Winston, 1969), p. 13.

[14]Thayer, *Farther Shores.*

[15]Leading contributors have included the Allen-Bradley Co., the Lilly Endowment, the Deering-Milliken Foundation, Patrick Frawley and his two companies, the Schick Safety Razor Company and Technicolor, Inc., the Charles Stewart Mott Foundation,

and the Sunline Foundation. Group Research Inc., "Finances-Right Wing," pp. 9–16, 27–31. This support correlates with the fact that Schwarz's "Crusaders" are a predominantly upper-status group. Wolfinger, "America's Radical Right," p. 17.

[16]Raymond E. Wolfinger, "America's Radical Right," p. 12.

[17]Ibid., pp. 10–13.

[18]See Chapter 2.

[19]Wolfinger, "America's Radical Right," pp. 9–47. The ideological typology rendered in this chapter is meant to be exemplary rather than exhaustive.

[20]Forster and Epstein, *Danger on the Right,* pp. 144–46.

[21]Group Research Inc., "Finances-Right Wing," p. 7.

[22]Ibid., p. 5. Note that this income pattern correlates with that of the other Fundradist organizations previously examined.

[23]*Homefront,* vol. 4, no. 3, March 1970, pp. 21–22.

[24]Jorstad, *The Politics of Doomsday,* p. 75.

[25]Forster and Epstein, *Danger on the Right,* p. 149.

[26]*Homefront,* vol. 5, no. 7, July–August 1971, p. 47.

[27]Thayer, *Farther Shores,* p. 257. The number of cards claimed by Bundy usually hovered around the one-million mark. Recently, however, the figure has shot up to seven million—perhaps a result of the recent acquisition of the files of the late J. B. Matthews of Joseph McCarthy fame.

[28]Ibid.

[29]*Homefront,* vol. 5, no. 7, p. 51.

[30]Jorstad, *The Politics of Doomsday,* p. 75.

[31]Thayer, *Farther Shores,* p. 257.

[32]The quotations are taken directly from a Church League letter which was sent to a large Philadelphia department store, signed by Andrew B. Hunter, Field Director, and dated 31 December 1968. Charles R. Baker, "Blacklisting," a Special Report from the Institute for American Democracy, 1969, furnishes a complete report of this activity. (The League also offers "special investigations" at $150.00 a day plus expenses and infiltration of various organizations at up to $200.00 a week.

[33]Ibid.

[34]Jorstad, *The Politics of Doomsday,* p. 76.

[35]Thayer, *Farther Shores,* p. 44 and pp. 142–46. The founder of the Rangers is Col. Wm. Gale, U.S. Army (ret.). He is pastor of his own church called, "the ministry of William P. Gale" and has been quoted as saying "Turn a nigger inside out and you've got a Jew."

[37]Group Research Inc., "Finances-Right Wing," p. 20. Christian Economics receives heavy financial support from the millionaire J. Howard Pugh.

[38]Ibid.

[39]The author attended a Beeny lecture in Media, Pennsylvania, in the summer of 1970. Beeny showed a filmstrip on the degeneracy of the hippie movement which included some rather risqué pictures of nearly nude women. The crowd made appropriate sounds of disapproval, and the lady in front of me moved to the first row for a better view.

[40]Group Research Report, vol. 8, no. 1, January 14, 1969, p. 3.

[39]The author attended a Beeny lecture in Media, Pennsylvania,

[41]*Newsweek,* July 13, 1970; *Wall Street Journal,* April 24, 1970.

[42]*First National Directory of Rightist Groups* (Sausalito, Calif.: Noontide Press, 1963), p. 37.

Chapter 9

[1]Eric Hoffer, *The True Believer* (New York: Harper and Row, 1951), p. 15.

[2]Richard Hofstadter, *Anti-Intellectualism in American Life* (New York: Vintage, 1963), pp. 131–36 (Hereafter cited as *Anti-Intellectualism*).

[3]In this connection the work of T. W. Adorno, *et al., The Authoritarian Personality* (New York: Harper, 1950) and M. Rokeach, *The Open and Closed Mind* (New York: Basic Books, 1960), are most helpful. For a listing of social scientific literature on research into types of thinking, see Rokeach, Ibid., p. 18.

[4]There were 350 of these stores operating in 1966. B. Epstein and A. Forester, *Report on the John Birch Society 1966* (New York: Vintage, 1966), p. 96.

[5]Although Society officials sometimes deny official connection with these stores, Robert Welch and other Society officers have

attended the openings of many of them; they stock material "recommended" by the Society and are extended credit for purchases from Birch headquarters. Ibid., p. 97.

[6]Ibid., p. 96. Corroborated by the author's limited experience.

[7]This claim is based on a visit to Reformation Books in the spring of 1970.

[8]George Thayer, *Farther Shores,* p. 227.

[9]One of the more interesting examples of Fundradist use of Birch Society literature concerns Faith Theological Seminary of Philadelphia. Carl McIntire is the president of the board of this institution. The author made three separate examinations of Faith Seminary's library during the 1969–70 school year. On each of these occasions the periodical shelves were found to be curiously bare of secular materials. There was, however, a striking exception. Large numbers of the Birch Society magazine, *American Opinion,* were scattered about the room. The only other secular periodicals present in any quantity were some curious tabloid newspapers devoted to alerting the world to the superiority of the Nordic peoples.

[10]This tendency is so pronounced as to generate incredulity in those not prepared for the experience.

[11]Quoted by Forester and Epstein, *Danger on the Right,* p. 108.

[12]Ibid., p. 70.

[13]Ibid., p. 83.

[14]George Thayer, *Farther Shores,* p. 221.

[15]Ibid., p. 222.

[16]An interesting example of this concerns Dr. Revilo Oliver, who was a faculty member of the Hargis "school" in Tulsa in 1962. In 1966 Oliver was pressured into resigning from the Society and its Council because of his allegedly anti-Semitic views. Ibid., p. 18.

[17]John Redokop, *The American Far Right* (Grand Rapids, Mich.: Eerdmans, 1968), p. 129, claims that the series was published in 1909. The authority for the 1910–12 time span is Frederick C. Grant, "United States Religion," *The Encyclopedia Americana* (New York: Americana, 1962), vol. 12.

[18]Frederick C. Grant, "Fundamentalism," *The Encyclopedia Americana* (New York: Americana, 1962), vol. 12.

[19]For a thorough account of the rise of Fundamentalism see Stewart G. Cole, *The History of Fundamentalism* (Hamden, Conn.: Shoe String Press, 1954).

[20]For an interesting account of this aspect of Fundamentalism see Richard Hofstadter, *Anti-Intellectualism,* pp. 117–41.

[21]Ibid.

[22]Hugh T. Kerr, "Protestantism," *The Encyclopedia Americana,* vol. 22, p. 686.

[23]This theological doctrine is derived from the doctrinal statement of the International Council of Christian Churches, Carl McIntire, president. It coincides very closely with that proclaimed by other Fundradists. For another example, see Edgar C. Bundy, *Apostles of Deceit* (Wheaton, Ill.: Church League of America, 1966), pp. 31–32.

[24]For a succinct literary account of this type of religion see John Steinbeck, *Travels With Charley in Search of America* (New York: Bantam, 1962), pp. 77–78.

[25]*Newsweek,* "The Preaching and the Power," July 20, 1970, pp. 50–55.

Chapter 10

[1]See John Redekop, *The American Far Right,* pp. 17, 183 for further evidence of this tendency.

[2]McIntire, WXUR, Media, Pa., July 30, 1970.

[3]Hargis quoted in Redekop, *The American Far Right,* p. 17.

[4]Carl McIntire, *Author of Liberty* (Collingswood, New Jersey, Christian Beacon Press, 1946), p. 116.

[5]Ibid., p. 14.

[6]Quoted in Redekop, *The American Far Right,* p. 17.

[7]See David Danzig, "The Radical Right and the Rise of the Fundamentalist Minority," *Commentary,* April 1962, pp. 291–98.

[8]*Newsweek,* July 20, 1970, p. 54.

[9]Eric Hoffer, *The True Believer,* p. 86.

[10]Raymond E. Wolfinger et al., "America's Radical Right," pp. 10–11.

[11]Carl McIntire's slogan of "No compromise, no surrender" is typical of this attitude.

¹²One of the clearest expressions of this position can be found in Fred Schwarz, *You Can Trust the Communists (To Be Communists)* (Long Beach, Calif.: Christian Anti-Communism Crusade, 1960), p. 153 (Hereafter cited as *You Can Trust the Communists*).

¹³Hoffer, *The True Believer,* p. 118, comments that this technique was emphasized by Hitler in *Mein Kampf.*

¹⁴Billy James Hargis, *The Far Left* (Tulsa, Okla.: Christian Crusade, 1964), p. 106.

¹⁵McIntire, "Author of Liberty," p. xii.

¹⁶Ibid., p. 115.

¹⁷Quoted in Redekop, *The American Far Right,* p. 98.

¹⁸Schwarz, *You Can Trust the Communists,* p. 61.

¹⁹Franklin H. Littel, *Wild Tongues: A Handbook of Social Pathology* (New York: Macmillan, 1969), p. 74.

²⁰Ibid., p. 83.

²¹Hoffer, *The True Believer,* p. 14.

²²Hargis, *The Far Left,* p. 5.

²³Quoted in Redekop, *The American Far Right,* p. 35.

²⁴Ibid.

²⁵Ibid., p. 36.

²⁶Quoted in John Adams, *Nation,* Sept. 30, 1961.

²⁷Quoted in Redekop, *The American Far Right,* p. 27.

²⁸McIntire, *Author of Liberty,* p. 3.

²⁹Ibid., p. xvi.

³⁰Ibid., p. 8.

³¹Ibid., p. 22.

³²Ibid., p. 57.

³³Ibid., pp. 3–4.

³⁴Ibid., p. 26.

³⁵Quoted in Thayer, *Farther Shores,* p. 232.

³⁶Quoted in Redekop, *The American Far Right,* p. 79.

Chapter 11

¹See Robert A. Schoenberger, *The American Right Wing* (New York: Holt, Rinehart and Winston, 1969), p. 2 and Franklin Littel, *The American Right Wing* pp. 77–78.

[2]McIntire, *Author of Liberty,* p. 13.
[3]Ibid., p. 26.
[4]Ibid., p. 109.
[5]Ibid.
[6]Ibid., p. 112.
[7]Ibid., p. vii.
[8]Ibid., p. 13.
[9]McIntire, *Author of Liberty,* p. 18.
[10]Ibid.
[11]Ibid.
[12]Ibid.
[13]McIntire, radio broadcast, June 29, 1970, WXUR, Media, Pennsylvania. "You can't separate God from the nation."
[14]Redekop, *The American Far Right,* p. 63.
[15]Edward Cain, *They'd Rather Be Right* (New York: Macmillan, 1963), pp. 199–200.
[16]Franklin Littel, "Social Pathology," a paper for a Seminar on Extremism sponsored by the American Jewish Committee, New York City, June 27–28, 1968, p. 4.
[17]McIntire, *Author of Liberty,* p. 12.
[18]The similarity of method and world view that various Radical Right groups share with their declared enemy has received much scholarly attention. Among the following selections the reader can find a representative sampling of such attention: Richard Hofstadter, *The Paranoid Style in American Politics,* (New York: Vintage, 1964), pp. 32–36, Forster and Epstein, *Danger on the Right,* pp. 20–24; George Thayer, *Farther Shores,* pp. 175–76.
[19]J. Allen Broyles, *The John Birch Society* (Boston: Beacon, 1964), pp. 14–17.
[20]McIntire, *Author of Liberty,* p. 7.
[21]Edgar C. Bundy, *Apostles of Deceit,* p. 44.
[22]Ibid.
[23]McIntire, *Author of Liberty,* p. xvi.
[24]This "religiofication" of virtually everything is a feature that many authors have noted. See Chapter 3 for examples.
[25]For an interesting account of how the principal impact of

early Christianity was to separate the state from religious ends, see Ernest Baker, *Principles of Social and Political Theory* (New York: Oxford, 1961).

[26]Quoted in Redekop, *The American Far Right,* p. 104.

[27]Arthur Koestler, *Darkness at Noon* (New York: Bantam, 1941), p. 79.

[28]Ibid.

[29]Edgar C. Bundy, *Apostles of Deceit,* p. 18.

[30]McIntire, *Author of Liberty,* p. 93.

[31]Fred Schwarz, *You Can Trust the Communists,* pp. 3–4.

[32]See Eric Hoffer, *The True Believer,* pp. 57–58, for an interesting aspect of this situation.

[33]Clarence Laman, *God Calls a Man,* (Unlisted, 1959), p. 38.

[34]Ibid., p. 45.

[35]Ibid., p. 38.

[36]Ibid., p. 41.

[37]See Arthur Koestler, *Darkness at Noon,* pp. 127–28.

[38]Eric Hoffer, *The True Believer,* p. 93.

[39]Sam Morris, radio broadcast, WXUR, Media, Pennsylvania, July 9, 1970.

[40]Beeny, radio broadcast, WXUR, Media, Pennsylvania, July 1, 1970.

[41]Hargis, radio broadcast, WXUR, Media, Pennsylvania, July 9, 1970. This is a close paraphrase of the Hargis statement. His meaning remains completely intact.

[42]Hargis, *The Far Left,* pp. 10–11.

[43]McIntire, radio broadcast, WXUR, Media, Pennsylvania, September 8, 1970.

[44]Quoted in Forster and Epstein, *Danger on the Right,* p. 106.

[45]George Thayer, *Farther Shores,* p. 231.

[46]Ibid., pp. 224–25.

[47]Ibid., p. 231.

[48]Forster and Epstein, *Danger on the Right,* p. 78.

[49]Ibid., p. 79.

[50]Ibid., pp. 108–9.

[51]Ibid.

Section 4

[1]For Hofstadter's own summary of these rubrics see Richard Hofstadter, "Pseudo-Conservatism Revisited (1962)," in *The Radical Right,* Daniel Bell, ed. (New York: Doubleday-Anchor, 1963), pp. 98–103.

[2]Examples can be found in the first three theoretical positions dealt with in this chapter.

Chapter 12

[1]Lipset was the first to use the term "Radical Right." He coined it to distinguish those who claim to uphold tradition while really attempting to radically alter the basic nature of the society.

[2]Seymour Lipset, "The Sources of the Radical Right," in *The Radical Right,* Daniel Bell, ed., (New York: Doubleday, 1966), pp. 307–72.

[3]Ibid., pp. 310–15.

[4]Lipset notes that historians have traditionally attributed the decline of the Know-Nothings to their ambivalence toward slavery, but suggests that the recession of 1857 may have been more important. Ibid., p. 310.

[5]Ibid., p. 314.

[6]Ibid., p. 310.

[7]Ibid., pp. 310–11.

[8]Ibid., p. 312.

[9]Ibid., pp. 311–12.

[10]Ibid., pp. 313–15.

[11]David Riesman and Nathan Glazer, "Intellectuals and the Discontented Classes," in Bell, *The Radical Right,* pp. 108–11.

[12]Ibid., p. 109.

[13]Ibid., p. 110.

[14]Richard Hofstadter, *Anti-Intellectualism in American Life* (New York: Vintage, 1963), p. 121.

[15]Hofstadter also characterizes this period as a time when attention turned from the individual salvation theme to that of the social gospel.

[16]Ibid.

[17]Ibid., p. 123.

[18]Hofstadter, *Anti-Intellectualism,* p. 123.

[19]In this connection the entire fifth chapter, "The Revolt Against Modernity," of *Anti-Intellectualism in American Life* is most informative, pp. 117–41.

[20]T. W. Adorno et al., *The Authoritarian Personality* (New York: Harper, 1950), p. 26.

[21]A pseudoconservative is one who claims to be upholding established order while consciously or unconsciously trying to abolish it.

[22]See both Alfred DeGrazia, book review, *American Political Science Review,* 44:1005, December 1950, and J. H. Bunzel, book review, *America Sociological Review,* 15:571, August 1950.

[23]J. H. Bunzel, *American Sociological Review,* 15:571, August 1950, p. 572.

[24]Richard Hofstadter, "The Psuedo-Conservative Revolt," Bell, *The Radical Right,* pp. 76–95.

[25]See E. A. Shils "Authoritarianism: Right and Left," in R. Christie and M. Jahoda, Eds., *Studies in the Scope and Method of "The Authoritarian Personality"* (Glencoe, Ill.: Free Press, 1954), pp. 24–49.

[26]Milton Rokeach, *The Open and Closed Mind* (New York: Basic Books, 1960), p. 14.

[27]Ibid.

[28]Else Frenkel-Brunswik, "Psychological Aspects of Totalitarianism," in Carl Friedrich, ed., *Totalitarianism* (New York: Grosset and Dunlap, 1964), p. 177.

[29]Ibid., p. 178.

[30]Ibid., pp. 178–81.

[31]Ibid., pp. 182–83, 195.

[32]Ibid., p. 196.

[33]Franklin H. Littel, *Wild Tongues: A Handbook of Social Pathology* (London: Macmillan, 1969), pp. 59–92 (Hereafter cited as *Wild Tongues*).

[34]Ibid., p. 60.

[35]Ibid., p. 64.

[36]This observation is *not* unique to Littel, has been noted previously and, the author believes, is quite true.

[37]Franklin H. Littel, *Wild Tongues,* p. ix.

[38]Hannah Arendt, *The Origins of Totalitarianism* (Cleveland: Meridan, 1963).

[39]Franklin H. Littel, *Wild Tongues,* pp. 72–73.

[40]D. J. Levinson, "An Approach to the Theory and Measurement of Ethnocentric Ideology," *Journal of Psychology,* 28:19–39, 1949.

[41]D. Katz and K. W. Braly, "Verbal Stereotypes and Racial Prejudice," in G. E. Swanson et al., eds., *Readings in Social Psychology* (New York: Holt, 1952), pp. 67–73.

[42]Milton Rokeach, "A Method for Studying Individual Differences in Narrow Mindedness," *Journal of Personality* 20: 219–33, 1951, and "Narrow-mindedness" and "Personality," *Journal of Personality,* 20: 234–51, 1951.

Chapter 13

[1]Herber Kohl, *The Age of Complexity* (New York: Mentor, 1965), p. 14.

[2]In most instances the Fundradists object to a secular government directing the individual but strongly suggest that their proposed theocratic state would have no such policy. This tendency is hinted at by their enthusiastic support of the government's efforts to root out "Communists" through Congressional investigations.

[3]Quoted in T. Wallbank and Alastair Taylor, *Civilization Past and Present* (Chicago: Scott-Foresman, 1956), p. 341.

[4]Max Weber, *The Protestant Ethic and the Spirit of Capitalism* (New York: Scribners, 1968), pp. 121–22, 162–65.

[5]Ibid., foreword by R. H. Tawney, p. 3.

[6]This suggests that the Fundradists' mythic Golden Age, mentioned in Chapter 2, may well have one of its roots in the Gilded Age of the last century.

[7]Winthrup S. Hudson, *Religion in America* (New York: Scribners, 1965), p. 302.

[8]Henry May, quoted in Hudson, Ibid.

[9]Ibid.

[10]The "Beecher Family," *The Encyclopedia Americana,* vol. 3 (New York: Americana, 1962), p. 427.

Notes

247

[11]"Lyman Beecher," Ibid., p. 426.

[12]"Henry Ward Beecher," Ibid., pp. 424–25 and Richard Hofstadter et al, *The American Republic,* vol. 2, (New York: Prentice-Hall, 1959), pp. 276–77.

[13]Hofstadter, *The American Republic,* vol. 2, p. 276.

[14]Quoted in Herbert Gutman, "Protestantism and American Labor," *The American Historical Review,* 72, October, 1966, p. 75.

[15]Quoted in Hofstadter, *The American Republic,* vol. 2, p. 276.

[16]Ibid., pp. 291–92.

[17]Ibid., p. 307.

[18]Ibid.

[19]Quoted in Gutman, "Protestantism and American Labor," p. 75.

[20]Carl McIntire, *The Death of a Church* (Collingswood, N.J.: Christian Beacon Press, 1967), p. 82.

[21]Edgar C. Bundy, *Apostles of Deceit,* p. 44.

[22]Timothy L. Smith, *Revivalism and Social Reform in Mid-19th-Century America* (New York: Abingdon, 1967), p. 9 (Hereafter cited as *Revivalism and Social Reform*).

[23]This definition is derived from a compilation of characteristics gathered during research on the history of Protestantism in America.

[24]Historians of religion commonly argue that the first wave of evangelicalism declined to the point of nonexistence after 1850. However, in Timothy Smith's prize-winning book, *Revivalism and Social Reform in Mid-19th-Century America,* we find a convincing argument that this is not so. This time span is based on Smith's contentions.

[25]Ibid., p. 8.

[26]William McLaughlin, *Modern Revivalism* (New York: Ronald Press, 1959), pp. 105–6.

[27]Norman Maring, Professor of Church History, Eastern Baptist Seminary, telephone interview, January 20, 1971.

[28]McLaughlin, *Modern Revivalism,* pp. 105–6.

[29]Ibid., p. 107.

[30]Ibid., pp. 105–6, for a typical example.

[31]Smith, *Revivalism and Social Reform,* p. 236.

[32]Ibid.

[33]Ibid., p. 235.

[34]Hudson, *Religion in America,* pp. 321–22.

[35]Ibid.

[36]Refer to Chapter 10, p. 210.

[37]The postmillennial evangelicals were frequently involved in crusades to save the nation through moralistic reforms such as prohibition. Significantly, several of the few surviving prohibitionists are now n the Fundradist ranks. Examples are Dr. Sam Morris of San Antonio, Texas, "The Voice of Temperance," and Alex Dunlap of the Conversion Center in Havertown, Pennsylvania. Moreover, Fundradists commonly denounce "dirty books," gambling, ordinary card playing, dancing, modern movies, and a whole host of similar activities that bear a direct relationship to the moralistic causes of the postmillennial evangelicals.

[38]These last beliefs are supported by the fact that their denial would involve questioning the quality of the American way of life and the suggestion that free will may not be a suitable explanation for human activity—two views the Fundradists hold dear.

[39]Hudson, *Religion in America,* p. 302.

[40]Frederick Grant, "Fundamentalism," in *The Encyclopedia Americana,* vol. 12, p. 163.

Chapter 14

[1]"Fear Shouldn't Guide Text Selection," *The Courier-Journal and Times,* Louisville, Kentucky, September 15, 1968.

[2]Suggested Books on Negro History Off School's List," *The Courier-Journal,* Louisville, Kentucky, Thursday, September 12, 1968.

[3]Ibid. The director acknowledged that Drake's letter originated this fear.

[4]"Fear Shouldn't Guide Text Selection," *The Courier-Journal.*

[5]Suggested Books on Negro History Off School's List" *The Courier-Journal.*

[6]Ibid.

[7]John A. Stormer, *The Death of a Nation* (Florissant, Missouri:

Liberty Bell Press, 1968). Stormer is better known for his best-selling book, *None Dare Call It Treason.* He has become associated with Carl McIntire in recent years.

⁸Quoted in Ibid., p. 156.

⁹Ibid.

¹⁰Ibid., p. 108.

¹¹Ibid., p. 155.

¹²Jorstad, *The Politics of Doomsday,* p. 110.

¹³E. Merrill Root, *Collectivism on the Campus* (New York: Devon-Adair, 1955) and *Brainwashing in the High Schools* (New York: Devon-Adair, 1958).

¹⁴Mary Ann Raywid, *The Ax-Grinders* (New York: Macmillan, 1962), pp. 136–37.

¹⁵Ibid., p. 137.

¹⁶Quoted in Ibid. Another textbook censor of minor renown is the late Verne Kaub, a long-time associate of Carl McIntire and author of *Communist-Socialist Propaganda and the High Schools* (Madison, Wisconsin: The American Council of Christian Laymen, 1953).

¹⁷See Section 3 for details.

¹⁸Quoted in Arnold Forester and Benjamin Epstein. *Danger on the Right* (New York: Random House, 1964), p. 105.

¹⁹Carl McIntire, *The Death of a Church* (Collingswood New Jersey: Christian Beacon Press, 1967), p. 70.

²⁰One particularly interesting example of the Fundradists' support for resistance to school integration occurred when Billy James Hargis began a cross-country tour with Gen. Edwin A. Walker shortly after Walker had led opposition to the integration of the University of Mississippi. Forster and Epstein, *Danger on the Right* pp. 83–84.

²¹KYW–AM Radio, Philadelphia, Pennsylvania, "News Broadcast," Tuesday, February 15, 1972.

²²*Group Research Report,* vol. 9, no. 5, March 9, 1970, p. 19. S.O.S. places heavy emphasis on interracial dating and related issues in its appeals for funds.

²³*Homefront,* vol. 6, no. 2, February 17, 1972, p. 6.

²⁴John C. Walden and Allen D. Cleveland, "The South's New

Segregation Academies," *Phi Delta Kappan,* December, 1971, pp. 234–35, 238–39.

[25]Ibid., p. 239.

[26]Ibid., p. 238.

[27]Walden and Cleveland. "The South's New Segregation Academies."

[28]Professor Allen D. Cleveland, Auburn University, telephone interview, February 10, 1972.

[29]Robert Anderson, *The South Today,* telephone interview, February 10, 1972. See also Robert Anderson, "The South and Her Children," (Atlanta, Georgia: The Southern Regional Council), a 100 page pamphlet.

[30]Dr. John Millheim, General Secretary of the American Council of Christian Churches, personal interview. (Dr. Millheim is now at odds with McIntire and this could affect the reliability of his comments.) Dr. Millheim also admitted that the ACCC was still troubled by a segregation academy sponsoring member churches and that he abhorred the dehumanization that it implied.

[31]*Group Research Report,* vol. 9, no. 2, January 20, 1970, p. 5.

[32]*New York Times,* May 14, 1971, p. 43, reports a similar "conservative" protest school movement among parents of Catholic school children. One such school was started in Kinnelton, New Jersey, by Dr. William S. Marra, a professor of philosophy at Fordham University. Marra believes that "any intelligent housewife is as good a teacher as most of the people working in our schools today" and that when the nuns "went professional" they "began studying witchcraft and astrology." He started Holy Innocents after sex education became part of the Catholic School curriculum.

[33]United States Supreme Court, *School District of Abington Township, Pennsylvania* v. *Schempp* and *Murray* v. *Curlett,* 374 U.S. 203 (1963).

[34]Robert Kotzbauer, "School Prayer Issue Goes On," *The Philadelphia Sunday Bulletin,* November 14, 1971, p. 4, states that "a majority, perhaps 80 percent, of the American people favor prayer in schools."

[35]Bill Beeny, "Bill Beeny's 1969 Question and Answer Book," (St. Missourie, Bill Beeny Pamphlet, 1969), p. 29, contains a typical Fundradist allegation of subversion within the Court. Beeny asked "former Communist agent" Kenneth Goff, "Is it true that the Supreme Court has a record of voting more for the Communists than for Constitutional Government?" Goff replied, "Yes, the present Supreme Court voted almost 100 percent for the Reds."

[36]Edgar C. Bundy, *Apostles of Deceit* (Wheaton, Illinois: Church League of America, 1966), p. 83, claims that at this time there were a total of 147 different amendments offered.

[37]Quoted in Robert Kotzbauer "School Prayer Issue Goes On," p. 4.

[38]Ibid., Kotzbauer erroneously attributes this particular "Project America" to Liberty Lobby. A phone call to the headquarters of the 20th Century Reformation in Collingswood on February 24, 1972, confirmed the author's opinion that "Project America" was an I.C.Y. effort.

[39]Jorstad, *The Politics of Doomsday,* p. 117.

[40]Kotzbauer, "School Prayer Goes On," p. 4.

[41]Jorstad, *The Politics of Doomsday,* pp. 116–18, points out that with 1964, a presidential election year, Senator Barry Goldwater supported the Becker Amendment while Lyndon Johnson remained uncommitted. The Fundradists regarded the amendment as vitally important and found Goldwater to their liking. Jorstad speculates that these twin factors accelerated the Fundradists' growing willingness to set "total separation" aside and work with their secular brethren toward political ends. Hargis was less circumspect than the rest in making this change and paid for it with the temporary revocation of his tax-exempt status.

[42]Edgar C. Bundy, *Apostles of Deceit,* pp. 83–84.

[43]Ben A. Franklin, "Pennsylvanians Lead School Prayer Revolt," The *New York Times,* Wednesday, March 26, 1968, pp. 1, 20.

[44]Ibid., p. 20.

[45]*New York Times,* November 16, 1969.

[46]Carl McIntire, *Christian Beacon,* November 20, 1969.

⁴⁷Ibid. February 19, 1970.

⁴⁸Carl McIntire, *Christian Beacon,* April 2, 1970.

⁴⁹Ibid.

⁵⁰*New York Times,* April 5, 1970.

⁵¹Carl McIntire, *Christian Beacon,* April 9, 1970.

⁵²This figure was estimated by the Washington Park Police.

⁵³This figure was repeated many times throughout the late summer of 1970 over McIntire's radio network.

⁵⁴*New York Times,* September 4, 1970.

⁵⁵Ibid. September 26, 1970.

⁵⁶James Morris, *The Preachers* (New York: St. Martin's Press, 1973), p. 228.

Chapter 15

¹Personal interview with Dr. John Millheim, March 1971.

²Ibid.

Index

Index

255

and Freedom Center, 93–94
Collingswood Church, 71–73
Hargis, Billy James, 87–88
International Council of
  Christian Churches, 82–83,
  89
McCarthyism, 84–85
resources and organizations,
  3, 4, 52 69–97
Schwarz, Frederick C., 88–89
similarity to Henry Ward
  Beecher and Russell
  Conwell, 181–182
"Twentieth Century
  Reformation Hour," 91–92
MacRae, Allan, 77
Methodists, 185–186
Miller, William, 185–186
Millerites, 184–190
Millheim, John, 76, 96, 198–199
Mitchell, Henry, 199
MOMS, 34, 54–55
Morris, Sam, 147
MOTOREDE, 50–51, 54–55
Myrdal, Gunnar, 194
Mythic Golden Age, 12

N

National Association of
  Evangelicals, 81
National Conference of Parents
  and Teachers, 37, 62
National Council of Churches,
  25, 62, 200–201
National Education Association,
  5, 17, 23–24, 27, 33, 62
National Education Association
  and Sensitivity Training,
  59–60
National Education Association

Censorship in Kentucky, 193–
  195
National Education Association,
  letters to, 48–49, 52–53
National Training Laboratories,
  59
NEA *Journal,* 24
Negro history books, 193–195
"New Deal," 83–165
"New Math," 4
Noebel, David, 47
Noebel, David, *Rhythm, Roots
  and Revolution,* 127

O

Old School Presbyterians,
  185–186
"100 percent mentality,"
  163–167
OOPS, 55
Ozark Bible College, 87

P

Paisley, Ian, 151
Pelley, William Dudley, 83
POISE, 55
POSE, 34, 35
Postmillennialism, 184–186
Prayer and Bible reading in
  public school, 11, 199–202
Premillennialism, 184–190,
  188–189
Presbyterian Church of America,
  71
Princeton Theological Seminary,
  70
"Project America," 200–201
PROMISE, 55
Protestant Ethic, 176–182

About the author

Gary K. Clabaugh is Chairman of the Department of Education at La Salle College in Philadelphia, Pennsylvania. He is also Center Advisor for Temple University's General Education Program for Teachers at La Salle. Born and reared in Pennsylvania, he attended Altoona High School and Indiana State University of Pennsylvania, where he received his B.S. degree in 1962.

In 1968 he received his M.S. from Temple University. He won the Ralph D. Owen Prize for achieving the highest graduate average in the College of Education. In 1969 he was appointed a Fellow of Temple University. He received his Doctorate in 1972. His dissertation was titled *The Fundamental Protestant Radical Rightists: Their Views and Influences on American Public Education.*

For three years he taught geography in Red Lion Area Junior High School, Red Lion, Pennsylvania. During this period he had a confrontation with the local Radical Right which motivated his study of this movement.

A member of many civic and professional organizations, he is also a Fellow of the Philosophy of Education Society, and a member of the national honorary education fraternity, Phi Delta Kappa.

This book, Dr. Clabaugh's first, is the culmination of nine years' study of both the national and international Radical Right. He has lectured extensively on this subject.